The Body "Knows" Diet

Cracking
the Weight-Loss Code

CAROLINE M. SUTHERLAND
author of *The Body "Knows"* — *how to tune
in to your body and improve your health*

Caroline Sutherland
Nutritional Consultant and Health Educator
Sutherland Communications Inc.

IMPORTANT CAUTIONS TO THE READER

This book is not intended to diagnose any condition or disease, provide specific medical or other professional advice, or promote the sale of any product or service. None of the information or suggestions in this book should be used without first consulting a medical doctor and obtaining the doctor's consent to do so.

This book is sold on the condition and with the reader's understanding and agreement that the author and publisher shall not be liable or responsible for any damage, injury or loss alleged to be caused, directly or indirectly, by the information and suggestions in this book.

Public figures whose names appear in and/or on the covers of this book are mentioned for purposes of identification and comment only. No affiliation, sponsorship or endorsement is claimed or implied.

When private figures are identified by first names in this book, the names have been changed. Any resemblance between the names used in this book to identify private figures and any real individuals is strictly coincidental.

SUTHERLAND COMMUNICATIONS INC.
1 Lake Louise Drive #34
Bellingham Washington, 98229

To order:
www.amazon.com • www.atlasbooks.com

This book is dedicated to all
my clients who have lost weight on
The Body "Knows" Diet!

Caroline Sutherland is an internationally recognized health educator, lecturer, workshop leader and author of numerous books and audio programs on health, personal development, and self-esteem. She is the founder of Sutherland Communications Inc., which offers weight-loss programs, consultation services and related products for adults and children. For the past 20 years, she has positively assisted the lives of over 85,000 people.

Caroline is a popular guest on radio and television.
www.thebodyknowsdiet.com

What People Are Saying About "The Body 'Knows' Diet"

"I have lost 50 pounds on my program from Caroline Sutherland. I walk 2½ miles a day, and my doctor says that my blood sugar, cholesterol and heart function are 'beyond perfect.'" Caroline, thank-you so much!"
— Cheryl Beckman, Warren Michigan

"I attended one of Caroline's seminars last year. It drew people from all over the country. Her wealth of knowledge was amazing. Her program has positively affected my whole family — my husband has gone down three pant sizes and as an added bonus, he no longer snores!"
— Bente Hewitt, Gilroy California

"As a registered nurse I was interested in Caroline Sutherland's information. It has helped me gain a new perspective on the health and nutritional needs of the patients in my care. I was impressed with her presentation, which benefited me not only professionally but personally as well. I am no longer on blood-pressure medication, have increased energy and have lost 35 pounds."
— Gary Leikas, Portland Oregon

"I have been on Caroline Sutherland's program for about six months. I have found the diet easy to follow offering plenty of food choices. I have had a significant battle with weight over the years and topped out at 165 pounds. I am now 133 pounds, feel great, have loads of energy and get lots of compliments."
— Rosemary Tate, Bellingham Washington

"I have lost 100 pounds on my weight loss program. Nothing can compare to how good I feel and my sense of accomplishment." — Pat Spindler, Windsor, Ontario

Caroline's program has changed my life. I began to revise my old eating habits right away. It has not been easy. Mostly I have discovered over these many months of yo-yo-ing, that I truly have been addicted to sugar. And I am convinced now.

Thank heavens for Caroline's strong advice or I may not have been convinced. But her love, sincerity, and strong desire spoke so deeply to my heart that I couldn't erase the new information she was pouring in for my own sake.

Caroline is an angel sent to me after so many years of prayers about my compulsive eating disorder. I thank her from the bottom of my heart."
— Shannon Peck, San Diego, California

"I attended one of Caroline Sutherland's weight-loss seminars. Without any expectations, I instituted her suggestions. Within three months, I lost 40 pounds, my joints are no longer stiff and I can think clearly. My family says I look years younger. I am so happy."
— Jean Eastman, Portland, Oregon

"Since I was introduced to your diet, I've lost 48 pounds. I followed your food-allergy avoidance program, eradicating Candida yeast and improving my thyroid function. You helped me demystify my body's processes. I no longer wake up with a stuffy nose and headaches, my body doesn't hurt and I have five times more energy than I did before."
— Mickey Thurman, Santa Cruz California

Contents

INTRODUCTION 11

CHAPTER 1   The Five Components of Successful
Weight Loss 15

CHAPTER 2   My Story 21

CHAPTER 3   Celebrities with Weight Problems 33

CHAPTER 4   A Look at Top-Selling Diet
and Health Books 51

CHAPTER 5   How I Came to These Conclusions 77

CHAPTER 6   Common Food Allergies:
Weight Gain and Fluid Retention 85

CHAPTER 7   Candida Yeast, and Food Cravings.... 103

CHAPTER 8   The Carbohydrate Equation............... 113

CHAPTER 9   An Easy-to-Follow
Low-Carbohydrate Plan.. 121

CHAPTER 10   Exercise.. 125

CHAPTER 11   Hormones 131

CHAPTER 12   Emotions and Weight Gain 137

CHAPTER 13   Getting Started on Your Program..... 143

CHAPTER 14   Typical Questions and Answers 147

CHAPTER 15   Clothes and Colors 173

CHAPTER 16   The Benefits of Losing Weight 175

CHAPTER 17   Overweight Children 179

CHAPTER 18   Testing Yourself
   for Food Allergies................................. 185

CHAPTER 19   *The Body Knows Diet* Food Plan......... 191

   Daily Food Diary.................................... 210

   My Food & Progress Log 211

   Supplementation 212

CHAPTER 20   Personal Motivation 215

CHAPTER 21   Carbohydrate Gram Counter........... 217

Food Families.. 221

Hidden Food Sources 225

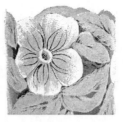

Introduction

Probably one of the saddest sights I see are overweight men and women poring over the diet meals in the freezer case at the grocery store. You know the "meals" I mean: small portions in fancy packages, minimal calories, no fat, no cholesterol — loaded ammunition. These meals are of little use to overweight people, contributing further to their weight problems — just because of what they contain.

Most people do not realize how simple it is to lose weight. Contrary to popular belief, losing weight is not about counting calories, weighing things on scales, measuring portions, or starvation. It's about knowing what the body wants and how it uses certain foods, even foods a person is allergic to, and translates them into cell tissue. I call this the great fat/fluid myth.

There are hundreds of diet books for sale. Every day a new "diet" hits the market place — the juice diet, the celebrity diet, the liquid diet, the grapefruit diet — on and on. Even the gastric bypass!

Every diet will work as long as the person is disciplined enough to follow it. But, funny how not one of these diets ever works in the long run or really catches on because each person is different. One person on the grapefruit diet loses 10 pounds, another doesn't lose an ounce. Why? With 60 million Americans dealing with some form of obesity — there just had to be a simple answer.

"The Body 'Knows' Diet" — Cracking the Weight Loss Code is the first book of its kind to actually spell out why weight loss is simple and easy to attain, and why no diet, despite all your valiant efforts, has worked for you so far.

I have had the privilege of working with thousands of clients over the past 20 years. I have seen successful weight loss in so many people that I needed to reveal the fact that we have been looking everywhere for answers to the weight loss question except inside ourselves.

I wanted to make this book really simple without burdening you with all kinds of scientific data.

The body "knows" — and is revealing to us moment by moment why we gain weight, retain fluid, have other health symptoms, and what we can do about it.

Ever since I was a teenager, I battled the weight problem. Up and down like a yo-yo over the years, I gained and lost over a hundred pounds until one day the secrets were revealed to me. And I never again experienced weight gain and that powerless feeling of being out of control around food.

I wanted to make this book really simple — without burdening you with all kinds of scientific data, charts, tables and menu plans. While there is always something good and useful in every book, I have seen so many diet books that are so over-loaded with this material that it can be impossible to find the "meat" in the message. So with this book, *The Body Knows Diet*, we cut to the chase, get down to business and show you what to do without a ton of scientific material, graphs or fat calculations to wade through.

If you want the scientific back up, take a look at some of the books I mention under suggested reading. These books can be useful references.

I encourage you to think of your new program not so much as a "diet" but as a lifestyle change; something that becomes a part of you. You see the wisdom in the five components of weight loss, you see the results, and you make the choice that this is the way you want to live. Believe me: after you have experienced the boundless energy and vitality that you will feel following this program, you won't want to go back — ever! Oh sure, you can visit the bread basket and the dessert table occasionally, but you won't feel great and then the choice to eat differently becomes automatic.

In this book, I have chosen to speak to you from the perspective of a person who has been there herself. I am someone who has experienced all the vicissitudes of the dieting and weight-loss game, the sadness and powerlessness that comes with starting a plan with the best intentions, failing many times, and finally to have triumphed.

Now it is my privilege to reveal these important secrets to you. If you want to experience freedom from the weight-loss battle, just as I have, without calorie counting, measuring, dieting, starving or exercising fanatically — read on!

Caroline Sutherland
SUDDEN VALLEY, WASHINGTON, SPRING 2005

Chapter 1

The Five Components
of Successful Weight Loss

For the past twenty years, I have been involved in food-allergy education. I worked as an allergy-testing technician for a medical doctor who specialized in Environmental Medicine. Multiple food allergies/sensitivities were very common among our patients. Because of this experience spanning many years, I have become very intuitive about people, their food allergies and system imbalances. I am a "medical intuitive": a person who has the ability to see beyond the normal levels of perception. My first book, *The Body "Knows – how to tune in to your body and improve your health* (Hay House), will introduce you to the fascinating world of medical intuition. I use this intuitive ability as a tool to understand why people have so much difficulty losing weight.

From the thousands of people I have seen, there is nothing that works more dramatically in terms of effective weight loss than the identification of common food allergies or sensitivities. I have perused every diet book and cookbook out there and they all seem to be missing this important piece.

There is nothing that works more dramatically in terms of effective weight loss than the identification of common food allergies.

Just taking a look at the diet meals in the grocery store is enough to make a person cry. How is anyone going to lose weight when the very diet foods that are being sold are loaded with allergy-provoking ingredients? Calorie reduced cannelloni Alfredo, for instance, contains two offending foods: wheat and dairy products. Plus it had chemicals, additives, corn derivatives, and salt.

Imagine $5 and 331 calories later that poor consumer, with the best of intentions, is going to be frustrated, still hungry and will probably have gained a few pounds because of what he or she chose from the diet counter.

My expression is not the first nor the last commentary on various diet plans or diet foods that point out their pluses and minuses. There has been lots of commentary and controversy surrounding these various plans — and there always will be — because "one size does not fit all," and while some of these diets are better for some, they are not so good for other people. The main thrust of my discussion is that all or most of these diet books or plans fail to or neglect to take into consideration the fact that some of the people trying to follow these diets and plans have common food allergies. I for one know what it is like to live with food allergies to dairy, and yeast in a world where most people can and do consume and add milk products, cheeses and yeasts with impunity into practically every conceivable food item but I also realize that not every one has the same problem with these foods that I do.

In short, my thesis consists of the notion that there are a lot of people on these diets who have undiagnosed food allergies.

Twenty years ago, food allergies and sensitivities were a relatively unknown field and something that probably most medical doctors today are more aware of than in the past due to the more dramatic and deadly peanut and shellfish allergies that have received more public awareness in the last number of years.

But food allergies and food allergy testing is still not a part of mainstream medical practice — most MDs' training in nutrition seems to have been rudimentary at best, so how can one expect them to know much about food allergies? My intent with this book is to point out that these well known diets, diet foods and plans fail to consider common food allergies and to help raise peoples awareness of this issue.

Most people do not realize that losing weight is very simple. Despite what we are taught, calorie counting, swearing off fat, starving or bending ourselves into a pretzel at the gym is *not* the way to lose weight effectively. We are admonished to "get real," to push ourselves away from the table, chew on celery sticks, or even go to bed hungry.

Oh yes, weight loss can be achieved this way. It can be done, but there is a much easier solution without the high price of deprivation and subsequent diet failure.

As a health educator, time and time again I have witnessed dramatic transformations in my clients from weight loss to clearer skin and reduced symptoms when they follow "The Body 'Knows' Diet."

I believe that through my own study, experience, and the observation of thousands of overweight people through the past 20 years, I have at last "cracked the weight-loss code."

I am here to impart to you the secrets of that code and to offer you the five important components of the weight-loss equation and help you to transform your life.

These are the five important components of effective weight loss:

1. *Food allergies*: most overweight people have food allergies or sensitivities — particularly to the common foods that they eat every day.

2. *Chronic Candidiasis:* most overweight people are afflicted with Candida or the Candida yeast syndrome, which can trigger tremendous cravings for starches and sugars. Candida is easy to correct.

3. *Excessive carbohydrate consumption:* carbohydrates (starches) quickly convert to sugar. Sugar converts to fat and is stored in the cells.

4. *Exercise:* let's get the body moving, stimulate the lymphatic system, tune and tone up muscles and fibers, increase the heart rate and feel better. Choose something simple that you can commit to every day.

5. *Hormone imbalances:* another major component in the weight question is hormones. Overweight people often have thyroid problems and related endocrine problems. Hormones require careful balancing.

These are the physical components, but there's another component — *emotions* — what are you *weighting* for? Many overweight people are bored with life and are waiting for something to happen. Often, they have a strong *inner child* and strong addictive tendencies, which constantly require food to feel better.

Everyone has emotional issues that they need to deal with. So many people are not satisfied with their lives, their work or their relationships and food is used to placate their deep inner yearnings.

If this is your story, then I have a practical answer: Use the companion CD included in this book — "Why Wait to Lose Weight?" — and re-script, reprogram or harness the mind to get behind your weight-loss program. As you play the soothing, relaxing CD each night, you will find in a very short time that your mind as well as your body will be galvanized toward your new behaviors and your weight-loss program.

Emotions not withstanding, in my experience weight loss can be achieved *purely* from a physical level when you follow the five components listed above. From now on, please don't dwell excessively on your emotions and don't blame yourself for your moods or past issues. Know that your body chemistry is revealing to you that you are out of balance nutritionally, which could be affecting you emotionally.

You will notice that within a few days of starting your program, your mind will become clearer and you will experience less emotional upheavals, which can be related blood sugar fluctuations or toxins in the body. So even though emotions are important (we cover them in Chapter 12), I believe that they are *not* the cornerstone of a weight-loss program.

Chapter 2

My Story

My battle with weight began in 1963 when I went
away to Switzerland to school. I was fifteen
years old. My father, a medical doctor took an international position with the World Health Organization
and I was transplanted from a peaceful, happy life in
the Pacific Northwest to the cosmopolitan city of Ge-
neva Switzerland. I weighed 108 pounds.

Imagine a 15-year-old girl, who has just left all her
friends and family behind, thrust into the middle of a
beautiful, vibrant city and a new school knowing no
one.

That was me.

I was at an all-time emotional low, dealing with
many changes and unfamiliar surroundings. So I pla-
cated my self with Swiss cheese — you know the kind of
cheese with holes in it — Emmenthal, as it is known in
Switzerland. I took a liking to this cheese and bought it

in great quantities after I arrived at the school. I would spend my pocket money on a kilo of Swiss cheese and a loaf of French bread. Sequestered away in my dorm room — I would eat the whole thing!

After several weeks, my clothes began to feel tight. I would write letters to my parents asking for more money to buy new pants, and bathing suits — I was popping out of them and I had no idea why.

By the time, several months later, I had spent the summer in the Swiss Alps eating cheese, chocolate and lots of French bread, I had gained nearly 40 pounds.

Thus began my battle with weight that lasted until the age of 38, when the secrets of my weight problem were revealed, liberating me forever from the vise grip of food.

Thus began my battle with weight that lasted until the age of 38, when the secrets of my weight problem were revealed, liberating me forever from the vise grip of food.

The Secrets Behind My Weight Problem

In 1983 I went for my annual physical. I was 38 years old and had experienced fluctuations in weight for 20 years along with a number of symptoms that had me quite puzzled. I was married and raising two pre-teen daughters at that time. I was also a freelance writer for a major city newspaper and glossy magazine. Like every good doctor's daughter, I went for my annual physical every year and I figured this check-up would be the same as every other one: blood pressure, pap test, a look in the ears and throat, and a few pokes here and there, and thankfully a clean bill of health for another year. I had been gaining weight, and had a few odd symptoms and had not been feeling terrific — not really sick but not really well either. As I lay on the examining table covered in a paper sheet, I discussed with my doctor the myriad symptoms I had been experiencing, plus my struggle to keep my weight under control. I also told her about the depression and feelings of overwhelm and anxiety.

Not only had I battled weight for at least 20 years, suffered from depression and at times anxiety. As if this wasn't enough to complain about, I went on to tell the doctor of my greatest fear. I had been bumping into things — the edge of a doorway, or catching my hip on a table edge or the back of a chair. I seemed to be losing my balance or my sense of perception. Could this be the dreaded warning signs of Multiple Sclerosis (MS)?

I thought for sure that she would say that these problems were all in my head. Surprise! I was met with interest and compassion. She appeared to have an immediate understanding of the problem.

After a thorough examination, she said that she suspected allergies to certain foods and a sensitivity to yeast could be the cause of all my weight problems and mood swings.

After a thorough examination, my doctor said that she suspected allergies to certain foods and a sensitivity to yeast could be the cause of my weight problems and mood swings.

Allergies! No way! Why, I had never broken out in a rash, hives, had an asthma attack or reacted violently to anything I had eaten, or so I thought. Allergies, I concluded, were for neurotics.

Interestingly enough, my doctor shared how she too had suffered from similar symptoms. She suggested that a special kind of allergist — a specialist in Environmental Medicine — could hold a key for me.

That was a very important day, and one that would shift me out of the world of fashion, change the course of my life, and lead me into an exciting career in health education.

My doctor referred me to a colleague who specialized in the treatment of food allergies, the Candida yeast syndrome, and environmental illness. In her opinion, it was unlikely that I had Multiple Sclerosis;

more likely, I had multiple food allergies and a sensitivity to yeast. It was worth investigating.

Tucking the name and address of the Environmental Medical specialist into my purse, I wondered what the next step would be.

It was November, just a few weeks before Christmas, and no one was going to deprive me of my shortbread, eggnog, and all other seasonal goodies that I looked forward to. We'd discuss the allergies later. I proceeded to eat and drink my way through Christmas that year. Then, when the last chocolate had called out to me to be eaten, and the last crumb of Christmas cake consumed, I was ready for my appointment.

Feeling more depressed than ever — puffy and bloated, with all the buttons straining on my blouse — I entered the allergist's office. The next piece of the puzzle was about to unfold. All of my symptoms were full-blown. There is no way that this doctor could have an answer to such a host of problems.

A very detailed history was taken, each symptom carefully noted, plus a list of foods I most frequently consumed, which was an unusual question for a doctor to ask. I had to confess that I had frequent cravings for sweets and bread. Testing was scheduled for the following day.

Environmental Medicine is a special branch of medicine that deals with the person's relationship to the environment. The approach is comprehensive and holistic. Everything a person eats, breathes, or comes in contact with can all affect one's moods, one's physical symptoms, or even one's weight.

Food Allergy Testing

The next day, during several hours of testing, I was to learn more about the effects of foods and chemicals on the body. In this testing area, I was fascinated to see a room full of different people react in different ways to the common foods found in the average shopping cart. This kind of testing, called intradermal testing, involves the injection of a concentrated amount of each allergen or substance under the skin, at ten minute intervals. The pulse rate is taken, reactions noted, and a wheal or bump at the injection site is measured. After ten minutes, each test is neutralized and individuals are brought back to normal so that subsequent tests can continue. The substance being tested is not revealed to the patient until that test is completed.

In my case, milk brought on stomach cramps, post-nasal drip, and a dry cough. My eyes became puffy and my face felt "full."

In my case, milk brought on stomach cramps, post-nasal drip, and a dry cough. My eyes became puffy and my face felt "full," as though I were retaining fluid.

Obviously the healthy cottage cheese salad that I ate every day for lunch was doing me no good. Wheat brought on a fuzzy feeling in my head and exhaustion; I could hardly keep my eyes open during the test. I was sad to think that I would have to give up making the eight loaves of bread that graced the family table each week. Bread was supposed to be the staff of life, but it wasn't helping me!

The testing continued. Oranges brought on a pounding sinus headache and pulsating temples. What would I do without my morning orange juice? Chicken — fatigue, arthritis in my hands, plus a raised pulse. Potatoes — fatigue, pain in my wrists, hands, and knees. One by one, all of the foods in my diet were being crossed off my list — what was left to eat? Coffee brought on a feeling of extreme exhaustion. I was well aware that caffeine made me hyper, but it was interesting that the bean itself made me feel tired. Corn gave me an instant headache, spacey feeling, and a stomachache. Corn? Why would corn be a problem? I so rarely ate corn except fresh from the farmers' market in the summer. But, as I was to find out, corn is everywhere: most packaged and canned products contain corn. Even baby powder, some toothpastes, and the gummed adhesive on envelopes and stamps contain corn. It's not so easy to eliminate.

Help! Stop! Things were going too far. But just as I was experiencing all kinds of reactions to common foods, there were other people in the testing room who were going through their own reactions as well.

Bill, a healthy but slightly overweight 35-year-old, was experiencing a runny nose, streaming eyes, and a red face from (he found out later) apples — one of his favorite foods. An hour later, when tested for wheat, he fell fast asleep.

Arlene, an attractive 30-year-old executive, broke out crying uncontrollably in the middle of a conversation. She had suffered all her life from depression. What could cause such a reaction? Eggs. She loved them, ate two for breakfast, and would even whip up an omelet for a late-night snack.

Colleen, an overweight nine-year-old, jumped up and down with hyperactive and aggressive behavior in reaction to sugar and milk. Ten minutes later, a neutralizing dose of the same allergen would clear her symptoms quite miraculously and return her to a normal calm little girl.

It was clear that all of us in that testing room reacted to the foods that we ate most frequently or the foods to which we were addicted.

Wheat, dairy products, and corn appeared to be the

worst offenders, affecting every single person in the room — but in different ways. I gained a new understanding of the phrase "you are what you eat."

It was clear that all of us in that testing room reacted to the foods that we ate most frequently or the foods to which we were addicted.

Then I was tested for common inhalants and chemicals — the things that we are exposed to in the environment. This was a revelation. Chlorine brought on fatigue and pulsating temples; even the tap water had to go! Formaldehyde brought on a headache and that spacey feeling again, as well as fatigue and an increased pulse rate.

Formaldehyde is impregnated into synthetic fibers. This was an important link for me because I always felt tired and developed a mild headache when I was researching my weekly fashion column. Many women told me that they found shopping exhausting. I am sure that it is not because of the overwhelming choices but probably because of the chemical emissions from all the clothing in the stores.

Surely the tests were finished. At this point my whole life, my diet and my career were being seriously challenged. How was I going to navigate my way through this information? It was hard to accept.

But we aren't finished yet: Just one more test — a yeast extract called *Candida albicans*. This test took 30 minutes.

> *Just one more test — a yeast extract called* Candida albicans. *This test took 30 minutes.*

Within ten minutes, the test brought on a dry cough and that old familiar feeling of panic and anxiety across my chest. A few minutes later, this turned into depression. Then my neck and shoulders became stiff and the numbness and tingling in my arms and hands became severe. All of my symptoms were being graphically reenacted with a drop of this extract injected under my skin.

At last, all that I needed to know was there in black and white. I almost cried with relief that here, finally, was an answer. These reactions indicated that my "healthy" diet and Candida yeast were the cause of my physical symptoms.

After a full day of testing, I was barely able to drive home because I had such a bad headache from all of those food allergy reactions one on top of another. But the decision was clear: I had to eliminate my favorite foods temporarily so that my body could recover from their toxic effects, and I needed to take medication to eradicate the Candida yeast strain.

Noticeable Improvement

Within three weeks of taking a specific herbal substance to eradicate the Candida yeast, and making the necessary dietary changes, I began to feel better. The pain in my neck and shoulders and the tingling down my arms had diminished. I knew I had made a breakthrough when I could turn my head, without pain, to back the car out of the driveway. I adhered very closely to the dietary restrictions for several months, which was no mean feat and added considerable stress to my busy life as a mother and newspaper columnist.

But my energy returned, I was no longer tired and worn out, and the great bonus was that I could eat as much as I wanted, and as long as I stayed away from *offending foods, I lost weight*. My battle with weight gain was over. Most days I felt like a 21-year-old. My skin became clear and my brain and memory returned to normal clarity. My temperament and my attitude toward life was one of joyous anticipation. This is how we are all supposed to feel!

Chapter 3

Celebrities with
Weight Problems

Now let's take a look at well-known people in our culture who have been battling weight problems often for many years and see if we can piece together the reasons why. Believe me, I have compassion and admiration for people in the public eye. Public figures are under a great deal of scrutiny. Weight fluctuations, relationships, career changes — everything is under the microscope. In discussing celebrities, I want you to know that these are my observations and perceptions only and are not claims or statements. I chose these people because we all know them and are familiar with their trials around the weight issue. For over 20 years I have worked as a medical psychic or medical intuitive. I can "sense" what is behind a person's weight problem. My goal in this chapter is to educate you so that you can see your own weight-gain story in the following cases.

OPRAH WINFREY

It's a pity that Oprah — loved and admired by so many, myself included — has had such a battle with weight. This woman is an inspiration to millions of people around the world, and she has candidly shared her weight challenges with her viewers. We have been right with her as she has gained and lost weight over the years.

Now, as a result of consistent exercise and careful eating habits, she is losing weight and looking wonderful. Why do you suppose she has had so many weight-loss challenges?

As an allergy-testing technician, I frequently saw African American people whom I termed Digestive Lymphatic Hormonal (DLH) types suffer weight challenges because of milk allergies and hormone imbalances. I sense that Oprah Winfrey from early childhood may have suffered from hormone imbalances, notably what is termed *sub-clinical low thyroid*. Low thyroid can cause a person to feel sluggish and to have poor fat-burning metabolism. Well-known celebrities whom I instinctively feel share the same problem are Whoopi Goldberg, Queen Latifah and Star Jones.

Oprah, in my opinion, may be typical of many African American people or Native Americans, Hispanic/ Latino people and Indian people can be similar in this regard. Native Americans and African Americans do not have milk or milk-based products in their cultural lineage. Thus they can be reactive to them because they lack the digestive enzymes to digest the milk products.

Wouldn't it be wonderful if we could educate young African Americans, Native Americans and Hispanic people to consider that perhaps food allergies or hormonal imbalances may be preventing them from experiencing optimal health, ideal body weight, greater self-esteem, or personal motivation.

Oprah Winfrey employs a wonderful cook named Art Smith. I sense him to be a jolly, happy, outgoing person, and he also appears to have a weight problem. I have watched him on television and have seen his cookbook — very interesting! Many of the foods suggested contain common allergens. Perhaps Oprah could be eating foods to which she is allergic — *without knowing it.* Allergic foods trigger histamine reactions; thus, weight gain from fluid retention. (I explain this in more depth in Chapter 6.)

I believe that Oprah, just like many African Americans, could be allergic/sensitive to dairy products. So a delicious squash soup with just a dollop of sour cream could trigger a reaction in just 20 minutes later, which could result in a couple of pounds of stored fluid! Personal chefs would do well to consider the food-allergy concept.

MARTHA STEWART

For years, millions of people have admired Martha Stewart. Imagine creating an empire of megalithic proportions from a small catering and entertaining business. She has a huge following.

Regardless of Martha's past legal challenges (and, by the way, she's looking wonderful these days), let's take a look at the "cookie of the week" gal and see why she may have a tendency to hang on to those excess pounds. Martha Stewart is what I would term a Central Nervous System (CNS) type. This refers to any Caucasian person with white skin and light hair. Central nervous system types have difficulty handling excessive carbohydrates and sugars. I have found that in my research working with thousands of people, that Central Nervous System types tend toward hypoglycemia, prediabetic conditions and even adult onset diabetes unless they are very careful not to consume excess sugars and sweets. Now in her mid-60s, I sense that Martha Stewart may be consuming too many carbohydrates, which quickly convert to sugar, and all those cookies of the week end up around her middle. At this age in life, being postmenopausal, hormone balance is probably also an issue. My suggestion, if she were my client, would be to greatly reduce carbohydrate consumption (which, from recent photos, she seems to have done), increase exercise and consult with an endocrinologist for specific hormone balancing.

If you're looking for a male who shares a similar profile look at Drew Carey, star of "The Drew Carey Show."

Also a Central Nervous System type, my instinct tells me that if he were to reduce carbohydrates and stop consuming offending foods, he would have an overnight drop in his weight that I sense is largely stored fluid.

DR. PHIL

Bless Dr. Phil and all that he is doing to educate the masses on successful weight loss. Dr. Phil has a huge following and keeps people at the edge of their seats while he deftly pinpoints key emotional issues that keep people from being all that they can be and losing the weight they need to lose. He is doing a great job motivating people to be responsible and make healthy choices. However, his programs instill the adage in his many viewers that weight loss is about "getting real." Weight loss can be achieved by "getting real." But from my perspective and experience, there are more important components than attitude involved in successful weight loss. Even Dr. Phil, delightful as he is, may need to lose some weight himself!

A few weeks ago, I drove past a huge billboard with Dr. Phil sporting a milk moustache — touting the benefits of milk as the ideal weight-loss beverage. But I perceive that Dr. Phil may be allergic or sensitive to dairy products. He and his wife, Robin, have created a cookbook full of unquestionably tasty and beautifully presented but possibly allergy-producing recipes. The recipes may be low-cal. and fat-free, but there's the cheese and, from my perspective, if you look at Dr. Phil there's a characteristic little cheese roll, ever so visible, around his middle. By the way: his son, Jay (just a gem), may also benefit from eliminating dairy products from his diet. If you look at him he's a little bit pudgy — nice guy — doing a great work of motivating teenagers, but in my opinion, the elimination of dairy products from his diet would probably ensure that he maintained not only his ideal weight but might also help him to have clearer sinuses as well.

AL ROKER

Here's a man who really took things seriously. Al Roker, America's favorite weatherman, has undergone gastric bypass (Bariatric) surgery. It was very successful, over 100 pounds lost, but in my opinion he may not have needed to go to all that trouble and expense. Why? Al Roker is a Digestive Lymphatic Hormonal type (DLH). Remember: DLH types don't tolerate milk or milk-based products because they do not have the digestive enzymes to break down the proteins found in milk. Dairy products, in some people, tend to affect the lymph and trigger histamine reactions that could contribute to fluid retention. Along with falling into this DLH category, Al Roker would, in my opinion, benefit significantly from specific hormone balancing, notably thyroid, to stimulate the endocrine system for improved mood, temperature and fat-burning metabolism. Now the trick for Al is to keep the weight off post-surgery. Food allergies should be given careful consideration. This can be done by following the guidelines that I have mentioned.

CHRISTINA SARALEGUI

Christina Saralegui is the host of "The Christina Show" on the Univision Network, the nation's leading Spanish-language television network. "The Christina Show" has been very popular for the past fourteen years. In fact, Christina Saralegui's show is the number-one U.S.-produced talk show on Spanish-language television in the U.S. with an estimated world-wide audience of one hundred million viewers. Wow — move over, Oprah!

Christina Saralegui, like Oprah, has suffered with weight issues. Christina is a Digestive Lymphatic Hormonal type. Many people with African American, Native American and/or Hispanic backgrounds fit into this category. I would say intuitively that Christina's issues are digestive: inability to handle dairy products, and lymphatic issues, leading to fluid retention, plus excessive carbohydrate and hormonal imbalances.

If she were my client, I would suggest some thyroid supplementation and a close look at bio-identical hormone balancing. According to her Web site, Christina was born in 1948, which puts her now into her late 50s — slap in the middle of the "hormone hornet's nest." I cover hormone balancing more thoroughly in Chapter 11.

At this stage in life, there is a tendency to put on weight around the waist. This estrogen dominance or estrogen-related fatty tissue responds well to a low-carbohydrate diet and careful hormone balancing. Carbohydrate reduction can have a dramatic effect on a skinnier waistline.

One of the pivotal pieces of the weight-loss equation is understanding the relationship between the Candida Yeast Syndrome and cravings for sugars and starches – possibly leading to addictive behaviors in other areas. Once Candida is under control, the cravings go away!

Wouldn't it be wonderful if Christina could pass this information along to her viewers who struggle with weight issues and uncontrollable cravings?

But what a beautiful, inspirational woman she is. Not even 60, she has done so much with her life to lift up the souls of her viewers around the world through her philanthropic work and her voice for good.

LUCIANO PAVAROTTI

Here is a man who is sought after around the world for his deep, rich voice. Pavarotti has opened the door for many of us to the world of opera and its rich treasures. Luciano Pavarotti loves life and he probably loves food.

Because of his Italian heritage, I would intuitively term him a "combination" type. This is someone who has central nervous system energies and sugar/starch handling issues as well as hormone imbalances, often characteristic of people who come from Italy, Eastern Europe, the Middle East, Russia, and parts of Asia.

If Luciano were my client – I would just enjoy his company. How could you influence a person whose rich cultural heritage predisposes him to enjoy food just as he enjoys everything else – with passion and joie de vivre!

But get ready, Mr. Pavarotti. The body knows, and it may ultimately reflect back what it is being served by, perhaps, adult-onset diabetes, a shortened life span, an ache or pain, large or small – but in the meantime, you are loved by millions just the way you are!

KIRSTIE ALLEY

Here is a striking young actress who has parlayed her weight in to a successful sitcom. Kirstie Alley is a gutsy, brazen and talented actress who was smart enough to recognize that the emotional roller coaster experienced by the average overweight person could be humorous, poignant, and capture a huge audience.

But I understand that she, too, has personally become tired of the tabloid press and its portrayal of the "Fat Actress," which is the title of her sitcom.

Apparently she has changed her diet and her lifestyle and has become a spokesperson for a well-known diet center.

Kirstie Alley is another central nervous system type. These people usually have white skin and light hair. Central nervous system types have great difficulty handling sugar and stimulants. In Kirstie Alley's case, my perception is that for the last few years she has probably consumed way too many starches and sugars, which have converted to fat in her system. Kirstie Alley is quite young. Usually such a young person does not suffer from hormone imbalances. If Kirstie Alley were my client, I would introduce her to the concept of food allergies and sensitivities, lower her carbohydrate intake, institute an exercise routine and probably suggest a Candida yeast eradication program. Caroline Rhea — the effervescent host of the "Caroline Rhea Show" and popular weight-loss reality show "The Biggest Loser" — is also a person who would benefit from the above suggestions.

From the male perspective, actor John Goodman fits the above profile.

In her "Fat Actress" sitcom, Kirstie plays the role of the obsessed over-weight person very realistically. This is often the powerful but sad truth of how an over-weight person lives – under the grapple hook of addictions.

In looking at her character, I would say some investigation into the need to placate with food might be quite revealing. When we experience loss, frustration or disappointment, the first place we turn for solace is the refrigerator. Kirstie Alley may be an independent, defiant and outspoken person, but now, success not withstanding, she has realized that it is time to get the physical house in order, and I commend her for doing so.

LARRY KING

Now you wouldn't think that the "king of talk" on nightly television would have a weight problem, but just take a look at him the next time you watch his engaging talk show. When the camera takes a side view, as it often does, check out his middle. Just above the belt line, suspenders and all, is that tell-tale jelly roll that tells me one thing: too many carbs!

Larry King, I am told, has had a heart attack. People who have had heart attacks are often encouraged to eat a fat-free, high-complex-carbohydrate diet and to stay away from red meat. I would suggest that if Larry King were my client he would benefit from following a low-carbohydrate program and to eat consistent protein, preferably animal protein as part of each meal.

Red meat, sworn off by so many as being "bad" especially for heart patients because of the amount of fat, might be very helpful, in my opinion, because Larry King appears to be a "full power on" kind of guy. I find that with many similar high-energy clients, red meat seems to "hold" or sustain their energy for longer periods because it is a very absorbable form of iron and B vitamins. Because Larry King is a CNS (central nervous system type) it could benefit him to have frequent meals and snacks that contain some form of protein, nuts or seeds and to be careful about consuming excessive carbohydrates.

SUZANNE SOMERS

Suzanne Somers is a well-known diet guru and she has written several popular books featuring low-carbohydrate cooking. And now she has a new book out on the extremely interesting subject of hormone balancing — a very important component of successful weight loss.

Low carbohydrate eating improves hormone function because it helps to regulate the production of the all-important hormone — insulin.

Because of her knowledge, insight and dedication, Suzanne Somers does not have a weight problem. But for all her knowledge and wisdom, in my opinion she may be missing one thing: All her cookbooks contain recipes with dairy products — Parmesan cheese, sour cream, and whipping cream!

The interesting thing about Suzanne Somers — and I say this with the utmost respect — is that several years ago when she was undergoing treatment for breast cancer, she announced to the world on national television that she had very cystic breasts. (She is now cancer-free for five years.) In my research and education over the past 20 years, I have learned that dairy products and caffeine can block the lymphatic system; thus, for some people, creating benign cysts in the breast or other parts of the body. Not only that, in my opinion, I believe that Suzanne Somers may be allergic/sensitive to the dairy products she recommends. After all, milk is designed for baby cows.

By eliminating milk-based products from the diet as well as caffeine, this would help the lymph to detoxify, thus reducing breast cysts as well as keeping weight normal.

Because I am involved in health education, I am interested in what happens to people and their health challenges. So I understand that following her breast cancer diagnosis and subsequent lumpectomy a few years ago, Suzanne Somers underwent liposuction to "even up" as she termed it, the area where breast tissue was removed to match her other normal breast. According to the media, she was soundly chastised for having this procedure, but that's *not* what interests me.

In my opinion she may not have needed the liposuction if she had known that the very foods that she encourages people to eat may be creating lymphatic blockages or weight gain not only for her but also for her many clients. By the way: on the subject of a blocked lymphatic system, try eliminating dairy products and caffeine from your diet and you will probably notice much less cellulite!

ROSIE O'DONNELL

Rosie O'Donnell has made a significant contribution to the gay and lesbian community, advocacy for children, gay adoption rights and numerous charities. She's a character who is loved by many. She's not afraid to speak up.

Although she no longer has her television show, I recall that there were frequent discussions about the latest and best candies, cookies, soft drinks and sweets. I am very sure this woman had quite a sweet tooth. Diets seemed to be the bane of her existence and she delighted in encouraging people to try her favorite yummies.

People who crave excessive sweets and starches may be dealing with a ubiquitous yeast — the Candida albicans yeast syndrome. Remember my story and how this yeast affected my whole body. Because of candida yeast, cravings for sugars and starches can mean that a person is often powerless to stop eating them, thus contributing to weight gain.

In my opinion, Candida yeast is one of the biggest unidentified problems in the weight-loss equation.

In my opinion, Candida yeast is one of the biggest unidentified problems in the weight-loss equation, and

I suspect that Rosie's weight problem could be linked to this yeast syndrome.

I recall a number of years ago, according to reports, Rosie took several rounds of antibiotics to arrest the infection in her injured hand. Unless a person is very aware of the need to re-colonize the lower intestinal tract with a substance called acidophilus lactobacillus biffidus, then Candida albicans yeast can get a foothold in the digestive tract. When this happens, the person can become tired and crave sweets. Candida is easy to correct. Just ask for a Candida yeast eradication kit at your local health food store, or order the Candida eradication supplement at the back of this book.

It is interesting to note that people who are dealing with Candida suffer from mood swings or emotional issues and often blow things out of proportion probably because of related blood sugar regulation problems. Rosie has been known to be quite volatile at times, and indeed it has been her strength, but I wonder if nutrition and body chemistry might also be playing a part.

ROSEANNE BARR

Here is a feisty, fiery, no-nonsense woman who tells it like it is and has blazed an important trail in relaxing the persona of the stereotypical female. Bravo! Roseanne Barr is an interesting case. I call her a combination type. This is a mixture of the Digestive Lymphatic Hormonal type profile and the Central Nervous System type.

So here, in my opinion, we have issues with sugar handling, conversion of sugars and starches to fat in the body and hormone imbalances perhaps including thyroid. This makes for an interesting profile when you add in Rosanne's colorful personality. Many people use excess weight to protect themselves from being vulnerable, revealing the truth about themselves, or really shining as they were intended to shine. In my opinion Rosanne Barr fits into this category. Plus she is a comedienne, a profession well-known for its diversionary tactics away from the truth of who a person really is.

All of this aside, Rosanne has the admiration of many people. She was one of the first to be vocal and to make a statement about being OK in an overweight body and encouraging others to feel the same way. Rosanne has made many attempts through the years to lose weight — including gastric bypass surgery. If she were my client and was able to implement "The Body 'Knows' Diet" and the five important components of weight loss, I believe that she would not have experienced these emotional vicissitudes or suffered the pain of being overweight even though it has served her character and career.

WYNONNA JUDD

I have strong intuitive impressions about this very talented singer and the reasons why she has a weight problem. Lately, according to popular publications, she has apparently been examining childhood issues. In my opinion, while these issues and unfulfilled needs can be a contributing factor in over-eating, I really don't believe they are the key in this case.

I understand, from reading about Wynonna's life from time to time in popular magazines that she has suffered from asthma.

As an allergy-testing technician, I saw many people with asthma in our clinic. Often people with respiratory problems have been on rounds of antibiotics with little relief.

If a person has taken repeated antibiotics, they can develop imbalanced intestinal flora and *Candida albicans* can get a foothold.

When a person has an overgrowth of Candida they often become powerless to resist sweets and starches, craving them incessantly.

When a person has an overgrowth of Candida they often become powerless to resist sweets and starches, craving them incessantly.

These beautiful and thoroughly good individuals, through no fault of their own, then succumb to the grapple hook of these addictions and blame their emotional issues and their childhood for something that in my belief is strictly nutritional, biochemical and so very easy to correct. Sad!

Another factor in asthma is the common sensitivity to dairy products, which can aggravate the sinuses, nasal passages and respiratory tract because dairy products can be very mucus forming.

The first line of treatment in our clinic was to take anyone with breathing problems off dairy products. When a person is sensitive to dairy products or any particular food, the immune system can become reactive and initiate a histamine response, triggering various symptoms as well as weight gain through fluid retention.

I recall reading an article about Wynonna Judd. In the accompanying photo, she was leaning against huge, cozy pillows and surrounded by several dogs. People with respiratory problems often have many environmental allergies, notably to cats and dogs, feathers, and airborne inhalants — including pollens and molds.

Because of my personal experience, I have so much compassion for anyone who is dealing with weight and environmental issues. I wish that I could reach out and speak with each one and reassure them that their health and weight challenges are not a mystery and there is a clear path that lies ahead.

Chapter 4

A Look at Top-Selling Diet and Health Books

Now let's take a look at some of the top-selling diet publications and programs and see why I believe that they still fail to communicate the whole truth to the reader.

I want you to know that, as an author, I have the greatest respect for anyone who writes a book. To sit down and to put pen to paper and see the finished work is a feat of strength. I have written several books. It takes time, patience, research, personal experience and passion to tell a story. Countless hours glued to the computer, time away from friends and family as each word weaves a thread and a concept designed to change the life of the reader. This is the intent of every writer. But when it comes to many diet books, sadly, I feel that they are still missing the key ingredients.

While every one of these books carries important

truths, very few of them come close to helping the reader with the five components of weight loss. They may cover one component — low fat, low carbohydrate, or yet another "get real" and get-motivated component — but overall, the truth, in my opinion, is yet to be revealed from any of these books.

But, overall, the truth is yet to be revealed from any of these books.

Sadly, as I leaf through each of them I realize that the general public is still in the dark, still kept from the secrets and still without the information that will help them to take off and keep off those excess pounds.

Here's why — every one of these diet books is full of foods to which people are allergic or sensitive– namely dairy products and wheat/flour based products. Eating allergic foods trigger immune or histamine reactions and subsequent fluid retention equals weight gain. I will explain histamine reactions and fluid retention more fully in Chapter 6.

As you read the following discussion of the books in question, I want you to know that each author is doing the best job they can with the tools that they have and that my opinions are based on 20 years of work as an educator, a researcher and an allergy testing technician. Experience tells me that there is another way.

DR ATKINS

Let's start with Dr. Robert Atkins' *The Ultimate Weight Loss Solution* — *the 7 keys to weight loss freedom* (Simon & Schuster)

A pioneer in the field of weight loss, Dr. Atkins battled it out in the trenches trying to convince everyone, including the medical profession and the American Heart Association, that lowering carbohydrates was the route to go in shedding excess pounds. Dr. Atkins won that battle before he died.

I will never forget consuming steaks and cheese cake for a couple of weeks when I was 35 years of age, only to end up severely constipated, a face full of spots and a five-pound increase in weight. Why?

Dr. Atkins was a big fan of *dairy products* — cheese, cottage cheese, sour cream and whipping cream. I am highly dairy allergic, and that diet affected my sinuses, made me stuffy and bloated.

Several years later, when I was tested for food allergies, the secret was revealed why Dr. Atkins diet would not work for me. In my opinion, Dr Atkins does not take into account common food allergies, mostly those to dairy products, and there do not seem to be enough vegetables in his program. I've often noticed that people who follow his program can become very dependent on various meal replacement bars, low-carb products, and processed foods that contain several allergenic ingredients and chemicals.

On the plus side, Dr. Atkins program has taught the public that a low-carbohydrate program can produce the benefit of lowered cholesterol, lowered blood pressure, and regulated blood sugars. Fat, according to Dr. Atkins, does not make people fat. So that's a good thing.

In my seminars, I speak to thousands of people who have been on the Dr. Atkins program. Some of them have been successful, some have not. Often because of excess dairy-product consumption, many people appear to me to be toxic, blocked or like concrete. I suggest that if they increase their vegetable intake and eliminate all dairy products from the diet that they will probably get off their plateau and continue to lose weight.

Another glitch with the Atkins program when people reach that plateau and stop losing weight could be a result of poor endocrine function or inadequate hormone balance — namely thyroid.

Hormone balance is an important component in successful weight loss. If you have not lost at least 10 pounds in the first 30 days of your program, look to the food-allergy component and hormone balancing.

Hormone balance is an important component in successful weight loss. If you have not lost at least 10 pounds in the first 30 days of your program, look to the food-allergy component and hormone balancing.

Get a blood test and seek professional help in this regard.

THE SOUTH BEACH DIET

Next we will look at the popular "South Beach Diet" by Arthur Agaston, M.D. (St. Martin's Press).

This is another low-carbohydrate program, but a little different from Dr. Atkins: more vegetables, more choices, and a meal plan that is a little more uplifting than steak and eggs!

But in my opinion, it still misses the mark. Why? Because it disregards food allergies. For example, the mid-morning snack for the first day is mozzarella cheese! The dinner on Day One is fine: salmon, asparagus and salad — but, oops, there's that dairy again in the vanilla ricotta crème dessert! The measured portions will probably help with weight loss, but as soon as the person returns to their normal eating habits I suspect that weight will probably pack on again.

SUZANNE SOMERS

I love Suzanne Somers. She's a gutsy, brazen, good-looking lady who has done a lot to further the cause of the low-carbohydrate craze. She is also a very success-ful entrepreneur rising from humble beginnings and challenging circumstances to become a highly creative and wealthy person.

Her popular diet books all use a variety of dairy products in her recipes.

During my days as an allergy testing technician I observed that most people who had weight problems were allergic to the foods they ate — the common ones with dairy products being amongst the worst offenders.

DR. PHIL

Dr. Phil has become a national icon. Made popular by Oprah Winfrey when he was her courtroom counselor during her "beef" trial in Texas, Dr. Phil is a no-nonsense kind of guy. He tells it as it is, telling the people to "get real" and to get with the program. His book, *The Ultimate Weight-Loss Solution — the 7 keys to weight-loss freedom* (Simon and Schuster), provides many important points designed to motivate the reader to get on board and change their lives. I am sure that many of them do. But, in my opinion, Dr. Phil may be missing some important nutritional points that could really round out and enhance his program.

Dr. Phil encourages people to have "mastery over food and impulse eating." This important point would be much easier if he knew and could discuss one of the five components of weight loss — namely *Candida albicans* yeast, which can create tremendous addictions and cravings for sweets and starches. These cravings, in my opinion, are not all emotional but mainly chemical and nutritional, thus easily correctable.

One of the ideas that Dr. Phil discusses is consuming foods you have to work at to eat. He calls them "high-yield foods" such as snacking on sunflower seeds or other foods that you need to work at to eat. This is a good idea. But what about suggesting that people just eat a handful of roasted or unsalted almonds, cashew nuts or sunflower seeds that you don't have to work at and that would satisfy just as well? Another "high-yield" food that he mentions is choosing whole wheat bread over white bread — well there's still an exposure to the second highest food allergy: wheat.

Dr. Phil's principle may not be useful, and seems to me to have nothing to do with "high-yield food" or foods that break down slowly, but rather choosing foods that don't trigger an allergic response: shelled, unshelled or otherwise.

Another suggestion he makes is to use fat-free popcorn. In my opinion, fat-free or loaded with fat, it makes little difference because corn is a very potent allergen — one of the big five! Corn, a high-carbohydrate grain, converts quickly to sugar in the system and becomes fat.

> *Corn is a very potent allergen — one of the big five! Corn, a high-carbohydrate grain, converts quickly to sugar in the system and becomes fat.*

As an allergy-testing technician, I've learned that corn is one of the key allergy-provoking foods; thus producing histamine reactions, fluid retention and subsequent weight gain.

His book and companion cookbook, written by his wife Robin, is well researched and comprehensive, but loaded with allergenic foods. For example: Day Three exposes readers to multi-grain bread — made from wheat, a common offending food — and then on Day Ten the reader encounters multi-grain bread for lunch, or yogurt (dairy product) for dinner.

A very good idea and something that would be useful to all of us with food allergies — perhaps these well-known diet plans and cookbooks could offer suitable substitutes for dairy products, wheat and the other common food allergens that so many people are suffering from — knowingly or unknowingly.

(Note: If you have any of these diet or cookbooks on your book shelf, leaf through them and try to eliminate the recipes with offending or allergy-provoking foods, or substitute non-allergic foods in some of the recipes.)

The saddest Dr. Phil TV show that I ever saw featured a circle of overweight people crying about their feeling of powerlessness over their weight problems. Dr. Phil, in his familiar style, admonished his guests to "get real" and to change the way they think. Nice idea — very commendable but not always possible for every person because of addictions and temptations.

I don't think it's necessary to pack such a punch at the emotional level when it was so obvious to me that these poor people were suffering from the Candida yeast syndrome and nutritional imbalances, adding to their emotional upheavals.

I wish that I could reach all the overweight people in this country and assure them that weight loss has very little to do with "getting real."

I wish that I could reach all the overweight people in this country and assure them that weight loss has very little to do with "getting real" but everything about following the five components of weight loss and seeing those pounds drop off without having to examine or to dwell excessively on their emotional issues.

JAY MCGRAW

Dr. Phil's son, Jay McGraw, has just written a great book for teens: *The Ultimate Weight Loss Solution for Teens* (Simon & Schuster). This is an admirable work. Imagine a young man barely out of school using his power, talents and writing skills to motivate millions of teenagers.

I really like how this book is laid out: big type, easy to read, and each section is highlighted in blue. Good job with lots of tips and motivational techniques — but there are those food allergies again! Pizza, hamburgers, and cheese are suggested fare for our overweight teens, according to Jay, albeit in smaller controlled portions.

But the same five components of weight loss apply to teenagers as well as adults. Teens will lose weight if they understand that the big five allergy culprits are dairy products, wheat products, corn, soy, and yeast, and to stay away from them for at least a few weeks until they see the difference. When they know the truth about certain foods and how these foods affect them, then they will be able to make the right choices now and in the future.

I've had the pleasure of working with many overweight teenagers. I met Winston at a seminar in North Western Washington. He was 13 years old and close to 300 pounds. He mother said that he was a chubby and happy-go-lucky child. Now at 13, he was having problems keeping up with the others in P.E. class and was constantly taunted about his weight. His mother and father were both overweight and they shared with me their many failed attempts at following diets not only for themselves but also for their son.

They showed up at my seminar accompanied by Winston. I wasn't sure if a 13-year-old would be interested in what I had to say. How wrong I was! Winston sat at the end of the front row, intent on listening to the elements of the seminar. At the break, I encouraged him to think about what he *could* eat, not what he *couldn't*. He was optimistic about the new food choices.

The family left that night with renewed hope, plus a bag of assorted alternative crackers and a jar of nut butter — just to get them started.

Ten days later, I checked in with the family. Winston had lost 10 pounds without trying. He was enjoying the new foods, he wasn't hungry, and his parents were leaving at that moment to buy him a skate board. His mother said: "This is the first time that Winston has lost weight without effort. We are all encouraged by this program."

EAT RIGHT FOR YOUR BLOOD TYPE

This is the work of Peter D'Adamo who suggests that the four blood groups — O, A, B and A/B — have certain nutritional requirements. *Eat Right 4 your Blood Type* (Putman) is a very popular book, and quite revolutionary. In my seminars, I am often asked what I think of D'Adamo's concept. Well, I am type O and, according to D'Adamo's research, I shouldn't be eating wheat but should be eating red meat. I have not eaten wheat in 20 years and I do eat red meat because it increases my stamina, but not because Peter D'Adamo suggested it. So I find for type O at least in my case he is accurate. But D'Adamo suggests that type A should be vegetarian, that type B can tolerate dairy products, and that type A/B can be vegetarians and consume dairy products.

This book, in my opinion, is another one that gives blanket solutions. There are no "one size fits all" universal solutions. Individual food allergies need to be taken into account. You would not believe the number of sick vegetarians that I see in my seminars, and many of them have been encouraged to follow similar programs that do not take into account individual allergies or imbalances. Be careful. If you are going to follow a program then you will know by the way you feel whether or not it is working for you. Trust your body. The body *knows* and it will reflect back to you with energy, vitality and excellent health if likes what you are doing, regardless of your blood type.

Dr. Andrew Weil

Here's a man who is a real pioneer. I have been very fortunate to have met many wonderful courageous medical doctors who have risked everything to bring the concept of complementary or integrative medicine to the masses. Andrew Weil is one such person. He's a wonderful researcher, a prolific writer, teacher and accomplished physician. His Web site is full of very valuable information, but if you look at his photo it seems to me that he has a weight problem. So if he's the expert, why isn't it working for him?

In his book, *Healthy Kitchen: recipes for a better body, life and spirit* (Harper Collins), which he co-author's with Oprah Winfrey's former chef, Rosie Daley, there's a section called "stocking the pantry."

Let's look, before you are even into the recipe section, where the red flags are raised!

They suggest stocking wild rice, millet and quinoa as well as bulgar wheat and couscous in the larder. I'm a big fan of alternative grains. Wild rice, millet and quinoa are alternative grains and loaded with useful nutrients.

But bulgar wheat and couscous are wheat. I'm surprised that Dr. Weil, with his wealth of knowledge, would not be fully aware of the numbers of people who have wheat sensitivities.

Reading further down the list under the heading of "flour," white and whole-wheat flour is mentioned for pastries and cakes. In my opinion, it is not a great idea to stock wheat or flour-based products in the house. When you are trying to lose weight and get healthy, it is best to leave the baking of fine pastries and cakes to others. Wheat is a common allergen for overweight people. I am not a puritan, but I am sensible.

If I started to bake cakes and pastries again, I would gain weight. I love a rich, sweet dessert — who doesn't? — but only very occasionally. I will pay a big price and feel tired and draggy the next day if I eat a sweet dessert, but I believe that you have to live in the world, and part of living life to the full is enjoying an occasional treat.

If I had a suggestion about the pantry, I would not include any flour made from wheat: white, whole wheat, non-organic, organic, and encounter it out in the world on only a very occasional basis.

In my own kitchen I have a small bag of sugar in the cupboard that I have had for 10 years, and a tiny ziplock bag of wheat flour (in my freezer) of which I might use 2 tablespoons once a year to thicken the gravy for my Christmas turkey.

So you can see the confusion even from the so-called health experts. Good information, nice pictures, tasty recipes no doubt, but when are they going to see the truth and impart it to us? I honestly suspect that some of the experts really don't know the truth — yet!

So you can see the confusion even from the so-called health experts. Good information, nice pictures, tasty recipes no doubt, but when are they going to see the truth and impart it to us?

THE CARBOHYDRATE ADDICTS DIET

Written by a couple of medical doctors, Rachel and Richard Heller *The Carbohydrate Addicts Diet* (Signet) suggests that people keep their carbohydrates low during the day, but relax their regimen at dinner, at which time they are encouraged to eat a "reward meal." This reward meal can consist of their favorite carbohydrates — even chips or dessert — if, believe it or not, all these items are consumed in exactly one hour. This is an important time limit in order to control excess insulin production, according to the Heller's research. This may work for some people if they do not have food allergies, blood sugar handling issues, and if their hormones are balanced. But most people who have weight problems have all of these issues.

When I look over some of the suggested items for the reward meal I can see offending foods in that list (cream, cheese, cottage cheese and flour), and I know that many people will probably retain fluid from the histamine reactions triggered by the common foods that the Hellers suggest in that one all-important reward meal.

We also know that when sugar enters the blood stream, insulin is released and, regardless of the time of day, that person is likely to be spiking an insulin response that may have the adverse reaction of fluctuating blood-sugar levels.

I am sure that many people have benefited from this plan, but I found the book too confusing. It offers food choices that not only trigger histamine reactions but continue the cycle of cravings and blood sugar issues because of the consumption of certain snacks and desserts during a period when abstinence from these items is best.

THE PERRICONE PRESCRIPTION

Dr. Nicholas Perricone — a dermatologist, anti-aging expert, and author of *The Perricone Prescription* (Simon and Schuster) — is the creator of the "Wrinkle Cure" program. His book effectively spells out the principles of foods that can cause inflammatory reactions in the skin, joints and other areas of the body. This book is more aligned with my philosophy and training than any other diet book on the market.

Dr. Perricone educates the reader to know and understand that certain foods (wheat, soy, corn, and yeast, as well as sugar, caffeine, and alcohol) can have an effect on symptoms, premature aging, skin tone, and mental clarity as well as weight gain.

For the most part, while his diet plan stays away from the common offending foods, he does suggest some dairy products with limited exposures — namely cheese or yogurt. This could cause a reaction in some people, especially in terms of weight gain and subsequent fluid retention, and also in people who live in moldy, damp climates and who may suffer from respiratory infections. Cheese and yogurt can be very mucous forming and may aggravate certain respiratory conditions. However, there is a lot of merit to this book and clients of mine in their 80s have successfully followed Dr. Perricone's program and have noticed an improvement in their digestion and arthritis symptoms.

JENNY CRAIG, WEIGHT WATCHERS, AND DIET FACILITIES

All of these centers and programs fill a need. They play an important role in motivating people to stay on track with their weight-loss programs. But again, as people understand the five components of successful weight loss with "The Body 'Knows' Diet," they will see that even these diet facilities encourage the consumption of offending foods.

Weight Watchers has had significant successes over the years in helping millions of people stay on track with their weight loss programs. People really respond to "checking in" and getting weighed at meetings and sharing their stories about pounds lost or gained.

But weight loss is not about "points" and "exchanges"; it is about staying away from food allergies.

Consider all those desperate dieters — searching

for answers and leafing through the pages of a recent addition of the *Weight Watchers* magazine. Judging from the pictures, recipes and information, readers are going to think that they are doing the right thing when they make the recipe for whole wheat linguini served in a sauce made from milk!

Then take a look at many of the prepared meals that people purchase when they sign on for a program at a diet facility: They are expensive (that's how these places make their money) and they are loaded with the five big allergens — dairy, wheat, corn, soy or yeast.

So how are you going to lose weight permanently on these programs?

It's probably not possible in the long term unless you adhere to their regimen. As soon as a person stops attending the diet facility and eats their own meals at home, they will gain weight unless they continue to eat the carefully measured, calorie-controlled portions of purchased or packaged foods.

Last year I had the opportunity to meet the director of one of these diet facilities. She was intrigued to learn more about my approach to the weight-loss equation. As she sat through my seminar she kept having "light-bulb moments" and could graphically see how the very "diet" foods that were sold at her facility could be triggering fluid retention and subsequent weight gain in her clients.

NUTRITIONISTS AND DIETITIANS

My mother was a dietitian. I grew up on home-made whole-wheat bread, yogurt and lots of cheese. I suffered horribly for years from constipation, respiratory problems and recurrent ear infections. If my mother had known about common food allergies as well as her wealth of knowledge about good nutrition, I would have been a much healthier child. Many people consult with nutritionists and dietitians. These people can be very knowledgeable about fat grams, calories, dietary requirements of vitamins and minerals as well as a wealth of important information but, they are still missing the "food allergy" piece.

Here's an example of a diet brought to me by a client who had been consulting a nutritionist:

BREAKFAST
1 meal replacement bar
½ cup berries or piece of fruit
1 cup skim milk
1 cup coffee or tea

I don't like the bar because it probably contains offending foods and chemicals. The berries and fruit might be better eaten later in the day so as not to spike an insulin response. Skim milk could cause a histamine reaction and consequent fluid retention. Coffee or tea can over-stimulate the pancreas, creating an insulin rise.

This is not an adequate breakfast in my opinion. It may be low in calories, but is it going to leave the client feeling energetic or satisfied?

SNACK
Dry-roasted peanuts

I would suggest roasted and unsalted nuts — use true nuts such as almonds, cashew nuts, macadamia nuts, filberts or pecans. Peanuts are actually a legume, a bean. They are higher in carbohydrate than a true nut, and dry-roasted nuts contain salt and other additives. Not a good snack.

LUNCH
1 slice of cheese pizza
2 cups tossed salad — lettuce, cucumber, tomato and green pepper
2 tbsp light ranch dressing
Water, iced tea or diet soda

This person's diet is doomed right here. If it wasn't blown at breakfast, it's completely tanked at lunch! In my opinion, this person is going to gain weight from this lunch and diet plan no matter how few calories it contains. Why?

You guessed it: multiple exposures to offending foods. The pizza contains wheat, yeast and cheese. The salad is fine, but ranch dressing is dairy-based. Dairy products are a common source of food allergen, and what nutritionist would recommend a diet drink?

SNACK
1 cup cubed melon, 1 cup berries or an apple

I don't see a problem with the fruit. But fruit is a sugar. Very soon after the fruit is consumed, the person will probably feel hungry again. Make sure dinner or at least a protein snack is not far behind.

DINNER
1 cup won-ton soup
1 serving of chicken with broccoli and snow peas
1 serving of fried rice
1 fortune cookie

Now the diet is completely blown. This is a carbohydrate-loaded meal. The only saving grace is the chicken and the broccoli. Won-ton soup contains wheat. Wheat is one of the big five food allergies. Snow peas are a high-carbohydrate vegetable. A serving of fried rice probably equals a full cup — about 40 grams of carbohydrate and a fortune cookie, a fun end to any meal, and though foretelling the future of the diner, contains that ubiquitous wheat. I'll bet that within half an hour of consuming such a meal, the person will be bloated and hungry again. No wonder people are confused and still have weight problems despite the advice of all the experts.

BLENDER DRINKS

People have found a smart and simple way to eat breakfast or have a snack. Herald the arrival of the "blender drink" or "smoothie." Many of these are pre-mixed drinks that are sold in cans or packets as a diet meal replacement. In taking a look at the ingredients, they may be rich in vitamins and minerals but the liquid portion of the "slimming" mixture is milk — either in powder or liquid form. So this kind of meal replacement, which would appear to be helpful because of controlled calories, may not serve the unwary dieter because of the exposure and possible allergic reaction to dairy products.

Whey protein may also trigger a reaction because it is derived from milk.

Take a look at all the ingredients in the blender drinks and smoothies that you purchase or make yourself — do they contain allergenic foods? Are they making you sick? Soy protein is a well-known protein powder used widely in blender drinks, shakes and protein bars. Soy is a high allergen and could be affecting you.

INTERNET DIETS

Good idea, but the ones that I have perused do not take into account common food allergies, the yeast syndrome, or hormone imbalances. Again, we are not supplied with the correct information to make a wise and individual diet selection. Plus, many of the Internet sites appear to be heavily commercially sponsored, confusing, and filled with conflicting information.

Take a look at my Web site, www.thebodyknows diet.com, and follow the online weight-loss program with me in an exciting and easy-to-follow video stream. It covers all five components of "The Body 'Knows' Diet" for successful weight loss, and offers testimonials from some of my clients, personal motivation, and related products for yeast, hormone balancing, and mental re-scripting. It's all designed to lead you toward your goal. Weight loss is not a mystery, and my mission is to help you to understand all the elements you need to put it together.

BARIATRIC OR GASTRIC BYPASS SURGERY

This is the last resort. Last year I attended a presentation by a health facility specializing in the bariatric (or bypass) surgical procedure. I was stunned and saddened by the number of people in the room, and I felt powerless to help them. Imagine if they knew the five components of weight loss?

It was evident, from my observation that every person in that room, even the instructor himself, suffered from food allergies. I saw a room full of people with hormone imbalances and everyone appeared to be struggling with the low self-esteem that comes with feeling fat, sluggish, out of balance, and desperate for answers.

Bariatric surgery is designed to promote weight loss by limiting the amount of food that the stomach can hold. This works to reduce food intake by causing food to be digested and absorbed poorly. During gastric bypass surgery, a small pouch is created at the top of the stomach where the food enters. The small intestine is restructured and the pouch is reconnected, limiting the small intestine's ability to digest food, allowing it to pass out of the body.

This surgery has been very useful and much touted by several celebrities. Dramatic weight losses of 100 pounds or more can do much to boost self-esteem and self-image while jump starting the weight-loss process. Yet there is a great cost: upwards of $20,000 and some serious medical risks.

But let's take a look at the post-bypass diet:

In the first week or two after surgery, bypass patients are encouraged to eat "mushy" foods and "crispy" foods. Dairy products such as soft cheeses and low-fat yogurt, instant breakfast made with milk and other dairy products are encouraged. For example, on the crispy food list: melba toast, or well-toasted bread is suggested. Oh no!

Wheat and dairy products are common allergens and can trigger immune reactions and subsequent fluid retention. Imagine losing 100 pounds and slowly putting it on again because of "offending food" consumption.

Several years ago, I had the opportunity of working with a well-known performer who had undergone bypass surgery. She contacted me because she was slowly putting back all the weight she had lost. As soon as I pointed out that she was consuming foods to which she was allergic, and she avoided those foods, she started losing weight again.

Bypass surgery can be a useful option for some very obese people who have tried every diet imaginable. However, protect your investment and surgical weight loss by staying away from "offending foods." Take the time to research a skilled practitioner and get your hormones balanced, which is probably why you have experienced your weight problems in the beginning.

In the next chapter I want to give you a little background and tell you how I arrived at my conclusions and why I believe that you will be successful when you follow the five components of weight loss.

Chapter 5

How I Came to These Conclusions

A fter several months of being his patient, the allergist who had been treating me for my allergies and yeast-related problems opened a door to a very exciting new career.

Realizing that I had good communication skills, was compliant on the new program, had a medical background, and was keenly interested in the whole field of food allergies and Environmental Medicine, he approached me to join his clinic and learn to be an allergy testing technician. This provided countless hours of experience and the knowledge contained in this book.

This opportunity to work in a clinic involved an intense, total immersion program, with much study and training — plus hours of work testing thousands of patients for multiple food allergies, environmental allergies, and hormone imbalances.

Our clinic attracted patients who had been chronically ill for many years — and who suffered from weight issues and chronic fatigue and who had been every where trying to find answers. It was very revealing to me that in a matter of a few months, often weeks, people who had been offered no hope elsewhere were beginning to turn around. These could be children with behavior problems, allergies, learning problems, obesity and many other specialized complaints.

The usual chronic problems for adult males and females were weight problems, headaches, fatigue, joint aches, allergies, and others. It didn't seem to matter what age the people were. Even a person in their 70s or 80s would make a dramatic health turn- around — it was all a question of time and of offering them the tools and information about their health conditions that they had been missing.

Because of my background as a writer and reporter, I naturally began to ask the patients questions regarding emotional triggers that could be related to their health problems or weight gain. Invariably a person would answer, "I was fine up until my father died," or "I was fine until I lost my job," etc. There always seemed to be an emotional component behind their illness or weight gain. Addictions to food that were emotionally based compounded the problem.

We had various innovative approaches in the clinic. We used sublingual (under-the-tongue) or intradermal (injections under the skin) tests to determine allergies and sensitivities. We used phenolics, which are core chemical elements or aromatic compounds that are found in foods, as well as vitamins, minerals, hormones and neurotransmitters.

For example, if a person is sensitive to a certain food, perhaps a grain like wheat (flour), they can be neutralized for the aromatic compound or the phenolic chemical found in that particular grain family. This neutralizes, or takes away the adverse effect that person may experience when exposed to the wheat or any other substance containing that core phenolic element. Along with avoiding the food itself for a limited period of time, phenolic neutralization seemed to be very effective. People with hormone imbalances could be neutralized for the core component of an appropriate hormone, thereby improving hormone function.

(Today, as part of my online weight loss program, special phenolic drops are available to my clients. These drops help to neutralize people for food allergies as well as assisting in appeasing or suppressing the appetite. See page 228.)

It was fascinating to witness dramatic improvements in people as they were neutralized for these substances.

Day after day, as I worked in the clinic I would marvel at these transformations.

The bulk of our clinical work centered around the identification of allergies or sensitivities to common foods, inhalants and environmental factors, and the treatment of the Candida yeast syndrome or chronic candidiasis.

The bulk of our clinical work centered around the identification of allergies or sensitivities to common foods, inhalants and environmental factors, and the treatment of the Candida yeast syndrome or chronic candidiasis.

It seemed that nearly every person who visited our clinic was riddled with this yeast. It was easy to treat and, almost as if by magic, when this yeast was eradicated, each person's energy returned, pounds seemed to melt away, and cravings subsided. This gave patients a chance to experience total health — usually for the first time.

The term *allergy* applies to a person who experiences a severe or mild reaction to a certain substance. If a reaction is very severe it can result in *anaphylactic shock*. At that point, the patient may need to be rushed to an emergency room or be given a shot of adrenaline to counteract the effects of the allergen in question. Bee stings, spider bites, nuts, shellfish and various other substances can cause this reaction in some people. But people may experience hives, inflammatory, respiratory or digestive problems from exposures to common allergens as well.

In this book I am referring to *sensitivities*, particularly to common foods.

Sensitivities imply that there is a delayed,
subtle or unidentified reaction with no known
cause from food or any other substance.

Sensitivities imply that there is a delayed, subtle or unidentified reaction with no known cause from food or any other substance.

With sensitivities, a patient may experience headaches, weight gain, fluid retention, digestive problems, skin rashes, etc. that, though uncomfortable in nature, do not require emergency medical attention and are therefore not considered to be true allergies. I will use the two terms — *sensitivities* and *allergies* — synonymously in this book.

My role as an allergy-testing technician involved the use of very sensitive, computerized equipment, which was a difficult system to learn, but I seemed to have a knack for it. This type of testing meant that we were able to determine, in a very rapid and painless manner, food allergies and sensitivities, organ, hormone, and neurotransmitter imbalances, vitamin and mineral deficiencies, pollen, inhalant and mold allergies, chemical sensitivities, metal toxicity, and body toxins.

The principle behind this form of testing is the premise that everything has a resonating frequency — the human body, plants, animals, foods, chemicals, and everything that is found in nature. All of these materials oscillate or vibrate at a certain frequency. This theory is based on *quantum* or *particle* physics.

From this type of testing we can determine if the samples, allergens, or individual substances are vibrating at the same frequency, or are in harmony with the patient or not.

The patient holds a part of the equipment and the allergy tester uses a probe to touch a designated acupuncture point on the patient's finger. Then each testing vial or sample is placed in circuit with the patient and, depending on several indicators, a positive or negative response is determined.

Most people preferred this form of testing over the sublingual or intradermal testing, which was laborious, expensive, painful, and potentially reactive.

This form of allergy testing is also great for children

because it's painless. In less than half an hour the patient is given a thorough and complete work-up and their results are available immediately. Because we saw about 50 patients each day in the clinic on which I performed about 200 separate allergy tests, I became very intuitive about my testing. Through this vast experience for the past 20 years I have developed many successful health and weight-loss programs.

REVIEW
The Five Components
of Successful Weight Loss

Now let's go over the five components of successful weight loss again and refresh your memory. In the following chapters, I will expand on each of these components so that you will have a better understanding of why to date you have had a battle with weight, and how from now on how you are going to win!

1. *Food allergies*: most overweight people have food allergies or sensitivities — particularly to the common foods that they eat every day.

2. *Chronic Candidiasis*: most overweight people are afflicted with Candida or the Candida yeast syndrome, which can trigger tremendous cravings for starches and sugars. Candida is easy to correct.

3. *Excessive carbohydrate consumption*: carbohydrates (starches) convert quickly to sugar. Excess sugar is stored in the fat cells.

4. *Exercise*: let's get the body moving, move the lymphatic system, tune and tone up muscles and fibers, increase the heart rate, oxygenate the brain and feel better. Pick something simple that you can commit to every day.

5. *Hormone imbalances*: another major component in the weight question is hormones. Overweight people often have thyroid problems and related endocrine problems. Hormones require careful balancing.

Next, we'll look at common food allergies and sensitivities and the role that they play in your quest for optimum health and dramatic weight loss.

Chapter 6

Common Food Allergies: Weight Gain and Fluid Retention

M ost people are not aware that the common foods they consume can be one of the most important contributing factors in regaining their health as well as in losing weight.

Remember that the big five food allergies are: wheat, dairy, corn, soy, and yeast. Add alcohol, sugar, and caffeine to that list as well.

Remember that the big five food allergies are: wheat, dairy, corn, soy, and yeast. Add alcohol, sugar, and caffeine to that list as well.

The following information will clarify for you, the affect of each of these foods on your symptoms and weight issues.

Many people suffer from what is termed an *addictive/allergic response*. This means that a person can actually be allergic to the foods that they crave, and must eat these foods in order not to experience withdrawal symptoms.

Many people suffer from what is termed an addictive/allergic response. This means that a person can actually be allergic to the foods that they crave, and must eat these foods in order not to experience withdrawal symptoms.

Food allergies (or food sensitivities) involve the immune system, which recognizes certain foods (particularly dairy products and flour or wheat products) as foreign invaders against which it must defend itself.

The allergen engages the immune system, which releases a chemical called histamine. A histamine reaction can induce tissue damage, inflammation and fluid retention. This fluid is stored in the tissue, rather like a filing cabinet. The body says, *I don't like what she's/he's consuming, so I'm going to store this in the tissue until I can figure it out later.*

Unfortunately, this never happens and the body can never figure it out later, because the person keeps consuming the same foods — which can be irritating the system — day after day. As soon as the person stops consuming the offending foods (which are usually the same foods that the person is eating every day) the body miraculously releases the stored fluid and excess water weight through urination.

As soon as the person stops consuming the offending foods, the body miraculously releases the stored fluid through urination.

Food-sensitive people tend to crave foods that release serotonin, the "feel-good" chemical in the brain. These are usually sugars and refined carbohydrates. These foods break down and quickly convert to glucose in the blood stream. Blood sugars rise, giving the person a temporary feeling of well-being. Then the pancreas has to release insulin to bring the blood sugar level down. If the blood sugar falls too low, this can result in feeling hungry, tired, edgy or dizzy. You will notice that your blood sugars become much more stable, and you have more energy when you choose to eat protein with your meals and snacks.

As soon as the American diet industry and the dieting population understands the simple concept of food allergies, then the entire industry will be revolutionized. I can hardly wait for that day!

Most people who are overweight mistakenly believe that certain foods that are low in calories will help them to lose weight. This is a big myth.

Dairy Product Allergy

Over and over I see diet books and weight-loss plans that push the low-calorie/deprivation concept, but guess what? All the recommended low-calorie foods are common allergens!

For example, one such low-calorie diet food is cottage cheese. Cottage cheese or any low-fat cheese is a staple in the diet industry. How many people start a diet with the best of intentions on Monday morning with a plate of low-fat cottage cheese and fruit?

Cottage cheese is a dairy product, which can trigger immune reactions. So the body recognizes the cottage cheese, low-fat or otherwise, as a foreign invader, mobilizes histamine, and the resulting fluid is stored in the body. This is why people have such a problem losing weight. As soon as people identify their food allergies, and stop creating histamine reactions, they won't be storing fluid in the tissue — thus they will lose weight.

Unfortunately, many people, especially those with weight problems, can be **allergic or sensitive to dairy products** in some form. Allergies to dairy products can contribute to other problems besides weight gain

— namely sinus problems (because dairy products are mucous forming) asthma, nasal congestion, respiratory problems, stomach aches (because of an inability to digest the milk proteins) "growing pains" in children, lethargy, irritability, constipation, diarrhea, headaches, lumps and cysts in the breast or under the skin.

> *As soon as people identify their food allergies, and stop creating histamine reactions, they won't be storing fluid in the tissue — thus they will lose weight.*

Dairy products are: milk, cream, cheese, yogurt, cottage cheese, sour cream, ice cream etc. — any product that is made from cow's milk. Nature intended milk for baby cows!

Butter is permissible because butter contains very few "milk solids" or milk proteins.

Eggs are not dairy products.

When avoiding dairy products, use:

Rice milk, almond milk, or soy milk are alternative milks. But be careful — these milks are really useful only for children (who choose to put milk on cereal), and they may contain too many carbohydrates for an adult program.

Soy cheese and rice cheese are available in health

food stores, but soy is a high allergen and rice cheese may contain too many carbohydrates.

Sheep, goat cheese, goat milk or goat feta may be useful alternatives, but watch for symptoms — particularly nasal congestion or fluid retention. Sheep and goat are a different food family and therefore may not trigger a histamine reaction.

If you want to lose weight, I suggest that you stop consuming dairy products, wheat products, sugar in any form, and caffeine for a period of four weeks and see the difference. If you are suspicious about corn, avoid it as well. Corn is a very common allergen.

Wheat and Flour-Based Products

Despite our belief that **wheat** is beneficial and the "staff of life," wheat and flour-based products such as bread, bagels, buns, pasta, cookies, cakes, crackers, couscous, etc. can contribute to allergies and many health-related issues. When I stopped consuming wheat, my arthritis completely disappeared.

Wheat sensitivities can be a factor not only in fluid retention and weight gain but gas and bloating, arthritis, fatigue, poor absorption, irritable bowel syndrome, diarrhea, or constipation. Wheat and gluten sensitivities are so common yet very people know it! Try taking wheat out of the diet for a few short weeks and notice the difference.

Because *wheat, oats, and barley* are all part of the same glutinous grain family, all three should be avoided to obtain maximum benefit.

Did you know that:

* One cup of cooked oatmeal contains 20 grams of carbohydrate.
* One hundred percent rye is usually tolerated by wheat sensitive people.
* One slice of 100% rye bread is approximately 25 grams of carbohydrate.
* Whole rye Wasa crackers are approximately 7 grams of carbohydrate per cracker.
* Spelt and Kamut are ancient strains of wheat and should be avoided because they too are wheat.
* The best way to improve your digestion is to remove offending foods and take digestive enzymes — available at health food stores.

Alternatives to wheat/flour:

* Rice, wild rice or brown is best. White rice or sticky rice has a high glycemic index and converts quickly to sugar.
* One hundred percent rye, amaranth, quinoa, millet and buckwheat (not a wheat) are all unusual, healthy grains.
* Potatoes, sweet potatoes, yams, squash and other starchy vegetables can be important alternatives

to the over-exposure to grains. These foods are unlikely to cause an allergic reaction but in excess, they are high in carbohydrate.

Always count carbohydrate grams. Try and keep the grams from starches and sugars (fruit, too!) at approximately 60 per day.

Corn Allergies

Corn can be a common allergen in overweight people. Why?

Corn in some form is almost always contained in baked goods or processed foods. Because corn is so sweet and breaks down quickly to sugar, it can contribute to excess carbohydrate grams, subsequent weight gain or blood sugar regulation problems.

Soy Allergies

Now let's take a look at your legume (bean) consumption.

Legumes, though tasty, can be hard to digest, contributing to that legendary gas and bloating. Peanuts and soybeans are also legumes. Coffee and chocolate belong to different *food families* (see p. 221) but they are also a variety of bean.

Soy is the fifth most common food allergy. Soy is a widely-used filler in the production of many packaged

foods. Soy can contribute to an increase in estrogen production. People who are overweight often have high
estrogen levels. Estrogen dominance refers to estrogen-
related excess adipose or fatty tissue around the waist.

The current popularity of soy consumption may not
be appropriate for every body. Leave soy and beans in
any form out of your diet for the first four weeks. Use
your instincts to detect which one of these foods could
be involved in your weight problems.

What are you going to eat? You are going to **eat
heartily** from everything else!

---

*What are you going to eat? You are going to
eat heartily from everything else!*

Imagine being able to lose weight without measuring out portions, starving and counting calories. What
a relief! Imagine being able to eat cashew nuts, avo-
cados, smoked salmon or goat cheese — foods you've
deprived yourself of for years — and still lose weight!
Miraculous!

Food Allergies and
Common Allergic Reactions

Certain people develop allergic reactions because
of sensitivities to normally harmless substances. This

can result in symptoms affecting any part of the body: breathing, digestion, depression, headaches, arthritis, skin rashes, or weight gain. The range and variety of items to which a person may become sensitive are endless. Sensitivities usually occur after repeated exposures to certain substances. Or the tendency to become sensitive to a substance can be inherited. For example: a person may have inherited an intolerance to cow's milk in infancy. Later in life this person could acquire an allergy to cat hair after repeated exposures to cats. New sensitivities may be added as a result of exposures or the environment. Most people are aware of their immediate allergic reactions, which can result in asthma or skin rashes when exposed to certain airborne inhalants, chemicals, or foods, such as peanuts or shellfish.

But there could also be a link, which is worth exploring, for people with unsolved chronic problems and weight gain. These are called *delayed reactions* or *masked food allergies* and thus reactions to foods or chemicals are not acute or obvious.

Look at Labels

It is easy to locate the most common food allergies. Take a look at the label of any bottle of vitamins. Right on the label it will probably say, "This product does not contain milk, wheat, corn, yeast or soy." This warning is given because these items, along with sugar and caffeine, are the most common food allergy culprits. Vitamin companies do not want to take a chance with their supplements causing allergic reactions.

Food sensitivities almost always occur from the items that you consume on a daily basis.

Food sensitivities almost always occur from the items that you consume on a daily basis.

Take a look at what you eat every day. Does this include dairy products such as milk, yogurt, cheese, ice cream or cottage cheese? These are all dairy products. Dairy products are the most common allergen and many people are sensitive and may have reactions to them — such as gas, bloating, bowel problems, stomach cramps, weight gain, fluid retention, puffy eyes, sinus problems and respiratory infections.

Are you consuming products containing *wheat*? Wheat is the second most common allergen. Wheat or any item made from a sack of flour, in any form, can cause problems with joint stiffness, arthritis, tiredness, exhaustion, puffiness, fluid-retention, poor absorption, bowel problems, heaviness and soreness in feet or ankles.

It is disheartening to see that in every popular cookbook and every women's magazine almost all of the recipes contain dairy items or wheat products in some form. No wonder people are gaining weight! There seems to be no escape from these pervasive factors. It's time to wake up and figure it out.

It is disheartening to see that in every popular cookbook and every women's magazine almost all of the recipes contain dairy items or wheat products in some form. No wonder people are gaining weight! There seems to be no escape from these pervasive factors. It's time to wake up and figure it out.

Corn is another common allergen. Corn in some form is found in almost everything packaged. Corn is usually a factor in people with weight problems because it converts quickly to sugar and changes to fat in the system.

Sugar, chocolate, and caffeine can trigger nervous system problems and should be avoided. I often see caffeine play a role in breast lumps or cysts (because it tends to affect the lymphatic system) and bladder problems as well as in pre-menstrual tension.

Many people are allergic to soy. For some people, soy is difficult to digest, can block the absorption of iron and B vitamins, and there is some evidence to suggest that frequent soy consumption may elevate estrogen levels. High estrogen is often a factor in overweight people. And there is some evidence to indicate that high estrogen levels may contribute to breast cancer and other estrogen related cancers. Soy is a legume, a bean. Many people are legume sensitive and have frequent exposures to beans without being aware of it. Coffee, chocolate, and peanuts are all beans in some form.

There are many common food allergies. Many people are allergic to nuts, particularly peanuts, which can be due to a toxic mold. Eggs, tuna, potatoes, corn, citrus fruits, shellfish, and some spices are common allergens. When it comes to these items, people are usually very aware of their allergies and already avoid these substances in order to prevent severe reactions.

As an allergy tester, we had a food panel at the clinic comprising over a hundred different food items. People were often fascinated by the selection. But over the years, and by testing thousands of patients, I observed that most people are allergic or sensitive to the foods which they *eat every day*, and not the strange, uncommon foods that they rarely consume.

Along with the identification of Candida yeast, which we will discuss next, probably the single most important factor in a person's health plan is the awareness of their food allergies. As soon the allergic or sensitive foods are taken out of the diet, most people usually feel a welcome measure of relief from symptoms, and they lose weight.

Food Allergies and Cravings

Very often a person may be allergic to the substance that they are craving. A medical doctor I know suggests to all her patients that they stop eating all the foods that they usually eat for one full week. She has researched the fact that in this brief period of avoidance most of her patients' symptoms subside. Let's take a look at where the cravings begin.

Many people are addicted to sugar. I have actually had people break down and cry in front of me when I suggest that they use an alternative to sugar for a short period, just to break the cycle. I have found that people crave sugar when they do not get enough protein. This is particularly true in the case of vegetarians who, unless they are very careful and are aware of protein combinations, tend to consume vast amounts of starch and sugar.

When sugar is consumed, the pancreas (an organ located just beneath the stomach, and responsible for the regulation of blood sugar) releases insulin.

When sugar enters the bloodstream, this insulin rise can trigger the desire in some people for wanting more and more sugar — almost as if the mechanism cannot be turned off. Stop triggering the insulin response and cravings stop.

A lot of people who crave sugar have rampant candidiasis. When Candida is under control, one of the benefits is that the sugar cravings subside. In a few short weeks, you will be able to walk past a bakery or a candy store with out being the least bit tempted. This has nothing to do with "will power" or "getting real."

People ask me how I manage my own cravings. Like many of you, way back over 20 years ago, I was addicted to toll house cookies, bread, and coffee. These cookies would literally call out to me from the freezer to come and thaw them out and eat them by the handful, which I did frequently.

Then I had the early warning signs of a serious illness. I had rampant candidiasis and its inherent sweet cravings. I also turned out to be allergic, or sensitive, to all of the substances that I continually consumed. In allergy testing, this is what is termed the *addictive/allergic response*. Food-sensitive people often crave the foods to which they are allergic.

Obese people can identify with the overwhelming power of food addiction. Food literally calls out to them and they become powerless over these irresistible cravings. Compulsive eaters continue to consume foods to which they are addicted many times in a day. These people, like the drug addict or the alcoholic, have no idea that their daily food cravings are based on a physiological need to prevent the withdrawal symptoms related to their food allergies. The solution is to stop consuming the foods that you eat every single day and eat heartily from all the rest until your system has ceased to respond negatively to offending foods and the immune system is given a chance to recover.

Food Allergies and Immune/Histamine Reactions

When people have food sensitivities, their body recognizes these substances as foreign invaders. The body reacts the same way it does to a cold, virus, infection, or bee sting. When stung by a bee, a person swells up and retains fluid at the site of the sting. The venom of the bee is a foreign invader to the body.

Similarly, as soon as a person ingests a food which is a sensitivity or foreign invader, the immune system mobilizes *histamine* and the person swells up or a part of the body may become inflamed as a result of this *histamine reaction*. Histamine is a substance that is released by the immune system to protect the body and the heart from the foreign invader or the allergic or toxic substance.

The key is to identify the foods that are foreign invaders to the body, eliminate them for a short period, let the immune system calm down, and stop initiating histamine reactions. There will almost always be an improvement in symptoms and there can be significant weight loss, by avoiding the common foods to which the person is allergic.

Once you discover your food allergies and I have outlined them for you – the big five, what are you going to do? Guess what? Eat heartily from everything else!

Chapter 7

Candida Yeast, and Food Cravings

Have you heard of the Candida yeast syndrome? One of the key elements, and the cornerstone of your desire to lose weight and experience optimum health, is the eradication of *Candida albicans* yeast. This strain of yeast — which occurs naturally in the digestive tract, skin, mouth, and nose — is present in the mucous membranes of all human beings. In a healthy state, Candida along with other yeasts and fungi exist in balance with normal intestinal flora, which is necessary for digestion, assimilation of nutrition, and the prevention of infection. However, under certain conditions, this yeast can increase rapidly and, in its fungal form, can overgrow the normal, beneficial bacteria. And because of our overuse of antibiotics, birth control pills (which can disrupt hormone balance and initiate food cravings not to mention our North American diet), our normal intestinal flora becomes imbalanced and this ubiquitous, ever-present yeast proliferates. Cravings for sweets and starches intensify the situation. Candidiasis is just as common in children as it is in adults.

Men are just as susceptible to Candida as women. This syndrome was very trendy in the 1980s. But an overgrowth of candidiasis can and does reoccur. Candida is just as important now as it was in the mid 1980s when William Crook, a medical doctor from Tennessee, wrote *The Yeast Connection Handbook* (Professional Books) and many other books on the subject. Dr. Crook, now deceased, is well known for his mainstream research and documentation in the area of candidiasis.

When I first read about Candida yeast, I was stunned and nearly cried when I read the case histories, particularly in women, and how similar their symptoms were to my own and those of many of the women that I assisted over the years.

I was stunned and nearly cried when I read the case histories, particularly in women, and how similar their symptoms were to my own and those of many of the women that I assisted over the years.

THE CANDIDA YEAST CYCLE

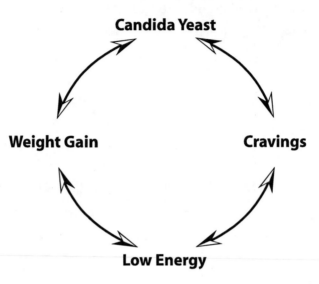

What I have observed is that this condition is almost always correctable. Over many years, I have seen the benefit of treating yeast in thousands of people with weight problems.

Candida albicans yeast can affect either sex at any age, including infancy. It appears to be more prevalent in women, probably because of the nature of their delicate endocrine systems. In adults this syndrome, and its inherent imbalances, is almost always diagnosed as a mental problem. The patient is usually told that it is "all in one's head" and is referred for psychotherapy. But the rapid disappearance of all symptoms when the yeast is treated illustrates the capacity of this fungus to be part of many serious imbalances.

Because Candida feeds on starches and sugars, it rapidly proliferates. Two common symptoms associated with Candida are *fatigue* and *sugar cravings*. Once the *overgrowth* of Candida is under control, these sugar cravings diminish.

Because Candida albicans is fed on starches and sugars, it rapidly proliferates. Two common symptoms associated with Candida are fatigue and sugar cravings. Once the overgrowth of Candida is under control, these sugar cravings diminish.

Thus the benefit is weight loss. Imagine stopping the craving mechanism — that power that cravings have over the body and our desire to eat and overeat!

Candida can also be involved in a myriad of symptoms such as: gas, bloating, constipation, weight gain, digestive disorders, headaches, fatigue, poor memory, mental confusion, learning problems, irritability, depression, respiratory problems, yeast infections, bladder problems, psoriasis, acne, low libido, hormone imbalances, toenail fungus, arthritis, autism, and it can even be involved in such serious illnesses as cancer,

Aids, Multiple Sclerosis, Chronic Fatigue Syndrome, lupus, and Alzheimer's disease.

I would suggest that if you have been diagnosed with one of these labeled diseases that you seek assistance in eradicating chronic Candidiasis immediately.

At the moment, although there appears to be plenty of evidence to substantiate its existence, traditional mainstream medicine rarely addresses Candidiasis. And because Candida is not always detected through traditional medical testing, it is difficult for allopathic medicine to recognize this yeast syndrome. Also because Candida Albicans exists within each person, its presence is often considered "normal" by the medical profession and therefore not considered to be a contributing factor in health issues.

But we are aware that fungus is in epidemic proportions, particularly in North America. Antibiotics, both from prescription medications and antibiotic use through the meat, poultry and dairy industries is a significant contributing factor to this yeast problem. Just look at the commercials on television for over-the-counter preparations for toenail fungus, psoriasis, dandruff, anal itching, and vaginal yeast infections. This is not a mystery. This is all about Candida albicans and its important link to these seemingly small but irritating problems. However, unless Candida is eradicated on the *inside*, topical skin preparations are only a temporary part of the solution.

Of all the things that I have witnessed in my clinical experience as an allergy-testing technician, there was none so dramatic as the beneficial effects of eradicating this tenacious yeast from the system.

Remember that Candida albicans yeast is fed on starch and sugar in any form. When people eliminate their heavy dependence on these items, this yeast cannot survive and cravings disappear.

Remember that Candida albicans yeast is fed on starch and sugar in any form. When people eliminate their heavy dependence on these items, this yeast cannot survive and cravings disappear.

In approximately one or two months, most of their symptoms dramatically improve.

An overgrowth of Candida albicans is not difficult to eradicate. But, as many people are aware, it frequently recurs and takes a lifetime of careful diligence to see that it is kept under control.

Many medical doctors rule out the possibility of Candida, because its presence is not always revealed in blood tests or stool cultures. Besides, Candida yeast is present in every single human being, so its presence is often discounted by the medical profession. I suggest that you locate a skilled medical doctor, naturopathic physician, or holistic practitioner who is familiar with Candida and can help you with this problem. There are many popular books available on the subject and yeast eradication kits and supplements are readily available in health food stores.

Most people whom I see have this yeast as part of their health picture. For instance, an overgrowth of Candida can make a person crave sweets and feel tired and most people that I see are exhausted. In approximately six weeks of following a Candida albicans eradication program, people are amazed at the return of their energy. Because Candida is fed on starches and sugars, of course it is an important component in overweight people.

This is a good time to begin using a natural sweetener like Stevia to sweeten beverages, or to sprinkle on a liberal coating of nut butter on a cracker for a midmorning or afternoon snack. I call that a "fake" cookie!

Chromium is an important trace mineral and can be useful to help with blood-sugar regulation and sugar cravings. Please refer to our appetite suppressant drops listed under helpful products, in the back of this book.

As well as all these useful ideas, it's encouraging to know that your cravings for sweets will diminish as soon as you stop feeding your yeast!

One of the more insidious aspects of this yeast syndrome is that Candida can attack healthy brain cells, thus contributing to memory loss. One of the most common complaints and fears that I hear people express to me is the loss of memory and the appearance of "fuzzy thinking." No, don't despair, this is not Alzheimer's disease or old age. This, more likely, is related to the presence of Candida albicans yeast spores, which circulate from the digestive system, through the bloodstream and these toxins can affect the delicate balance of the neurological system. After several months of treatment (because I have witnessed this for myself) as the body is detoxified, brain cells can regenerate.

This is how Candida yeast can affect people on the physical level. Now let's look at yeasts and fungi at a deeper level and see how they relate to a person's health.

Imagine that you are taking a walk in a forest, and you notice a tall, beautiful tree with a sturdy trunk and branches full of healthy, prolific foliage. Now imagine that you are looking down at the base of the tree and you see what looks like several white dinner plates all joined together, hanging off the side of the trunk. This is a fungus. The tree becomes the host to the fungus which lives off the tree, eventually robbing the tree of its vitality. This is the beginning of death for the tree.

So it is true in the case of the human being. A person with Candida is just like a tree in the forest. He or she becomes the host to the yeast or fungus, which lives inside him. Candida albicans in an overgrowth state is the beginning of the death and decay process in the human being and must be kept alive through the addictions to sweets of any kind in order to survive. Like a tree in the forest we do not want to fall before our time.

I find it ironical that the very substance — the sweet taste, is actually the element that we crave in our work and relationships. This sweetness in the form of sugar is consumed to excess, when the sweetness of fulfillment in life is missing, ultimately accelerating the body's breakdown and decay process.

When Candida Albicans yeast is present, the body's immunity and natural defenses become compromised and the system eventually breaks down and falls prey to the organisms, which live inside it.

The solution lies in building up the immune system with positive thoughts and actions and the reduction of sugars and excessive carbohydrates that feed Candida yeast.

Next we will take a look at the third component of successful weight loss — the carbohydrate equation.

Chapter 8

The Carbohydrate Equation

After you have identified all your food sensitivities and have eliminated them for approximately 30 days, the next step is to analyze your carbohydrate or starch intake. There are several popular books on the market describing the low-carbohydrate diet. These books can be a very useful education about how cholesterol is formed, how a low-carbohydrate diet can lower blood pressure, and help diabetic and pre-diabetic conditions.

But there are some problems inherent in the low-carbohydrate problem. One, there is too much emphasis on the consumption of protein, not enough emphasis on the consumption of vegetables or fruit, and too many processed and chemically laden snack items are encouraged. In the long-term, even though people can be very successful on a low-carbohydrate program, it can lead to an over-loaded liver and gall bladder and to some long-term poor eating habits.

The basic principal of the low-carbohydrate program is that you do not eat starches such as breads, pasta, cakes, cookies, popcorn, rice or potatoes in excess.

The basic principal of the low-carbohydrate program is that you do not eat starches such as breads, pasta, cakes, cookies, popcorn, rice or potatoes in excess.

A low-carbohydrate program suggests that you consume approximately 30 grams of carbohydrate for the first two weeks and sixty grams after that. This is called the "induction phase." But, I find that sixty grams of carbohydrate per day from the onset of a low carbohydrate program is a more manageable amount. Now you *are* counting.

If you are overweight by 20 pounds or more, and you are following a strict low-carbohydrate program you might want to consider taking a potassium supplement for the first two weeks of your program. If carbohydrate consumption is too low, the body can lose potassium resulting in fatigue, discomfort and heaviness in the legs. If this applies to you, I suggest that you take 1 potassium capsule (approx. 100mg) with breakfast and dinner for about 2 weeks and these symptoms should subside. Potassium capsules are available at your health food store. Potassium is a mineral related to electrolyte balance, therefore it is important not to continue potassium supplementation beyond the initial two-week period.

A low carbohydrate program focuses on the consumption of animal protein, or proteins in the form of beans, legumes, nuts and seeds, as well as plenty of vegetables and some fruit in moderation. Portions of the above foods are not limited, only carbohydrates (starches and sugars).

Be sure and eliminate foods to which you suspect you are sensitive before you begin, and always drink plenty of water.

Remember the big five food sensitivities are:
- Wheat
- Dairy
- Corn
- Soy
- Yeast

Add alcohol, sugar and caffeine to the list!

Alcohol and sugar are high in carbohydrates. Caffeine can be toxic to the body as well as stress the pancreas, liver or heart.

Here is the basic principle of a low-carbohydrate plan.

Let's say that you eat two whole grain muffins for breakfast — very healthy, right? After all, they are loaded with fiber, honey, dried fruit, and molasses. As soon as you start eating those muffins, they begin to convert to sugar in the digestive system. In less than an hour there is approximately one cup of sugar speeding around in your bloodstream. Then the pancreas, the organ that regulates blood sugar, goes to work and releases a substance called insulin to take care of this rise in blood sugar — the result of the two muffins.

At the same time that the pancreas is taking care of the rise in blood sugar, it also gives a message to the liver to create cholesterol in the same amount. The cholesterol is stored in the body unless it is used up in exertion (exercise). The secret behind the low-carbohydrate diet is not to initiate a strong insulin response from the pancreas. This way the pancreas is not overworked and constantly releasing insulin, nor is it constantly giving messages to the liver to create cholesterol.

When there is very little sugar in the blood, cravings appear to subside and the body uses up fat stores for fuel.

This plan can be very effective. Not only do people have more energy on a low carbohydrate program, because they are not consuming sugars and excessive

starches, but they tend to lose weight, lower cholesterol and blood pressure, and sometimes even lower or
discontinue diabetes medication.

Pity all those poor people who have been avoiding
fats and animal proteins — neither of which trigger an
insulin response — and consuming excessive amounts
of carbohydrate — which *does* trigger an insulin response — in an effort to lose weight.

With all due respect to the low-carbohydrate diet
books that are available, they are all *missing* one important element: food allergies and sensitivities. Almost all
of these books encourage people to eat cream, cheese,
sour cream and cottage cheese in liberal amounts.

Recently there has been a big change in the food
industry because of the low-carb craze — but are they
getting it? NO!

*Recently there has been a big change in the
food industry because of the low-carb craze
— but are they getting it? NO!*

One well-known food chain is advertising the "controlled carb — whole wheat wrap" instead of a bun.
Big joke.

All the advertising about low carb bread and low-carb
pasta is very interesting, but guess what: it's still being

made from wheat flour. Wheat based products made from any kind of wheat flour will trigger a histamine reaction in an over-weight person and that person will retain fluid as a result of eating that low-carb, wheat bread.

Find out what is in the low carb bread. If it's wheat — forget it!

Have a rice cake or a rice cracker instead, or a yummy grain like quinoa. You won't be triggering a histamine reaction with rice and, consequently, you won't be retaining fluid.

Remember, in my experience, the number one food sensitivity for most people with weight problems and assorted health problems is dairy products. It's baffling that no one has figured out this obvious tie-in.

It's baffling that no one has figured out this obvious tie-in.

When people have been on a low-carbohydrate diet and have reached a plateau or have not lost a significant amount of weight, I encourage them to avoid dairy products for several weeks. Usually this will be the linchpin and the weight starts dropping off again. A low-carbohydrate plan can be another very useful part of the weight-loss equation.

When following a low-carbohydrate plan, it can be

useful to avoid caffeine. Caffeine stimulates a temporary surge in blood sugar, which can be followed by an over-production of insulin and consequent low-blood sugar downward spiral. An excellent reference for following a low-carbohydrate plan is *Protein Power* (Bantam Doubleday Dell) by a medical doctor husband and wife team, Mary Dan and Michael Eades.

Remember to take into account your own personal food allergies and sensitivities before following any dietary plan and always consult with your medical doctor when following any diet plan in case medications need to be adjusted.

Plan to keep your carbohydrate intake at approximately 60 grams per day. It can be helpful not to take fruit or carbohydrate at breakfast and lunch, so that insulin levels are not increased during those times, and there is no subsequent drop in blood sugar levels. Save the carbohydrates for dinner, when a drop in blood sugar and energy will not affect late day activities. Many people find that if they eat carbohydrate — even fruit or a small amount of starch — at breakfast or lunch, they continue to crave these sweets and starches for the rest of the day. Experiment with this yourself. Your body is the laboratory and it will show you the effect of what you are doing.

I do *not* calculate the carbohydrate in vegetables as part of the 60 gram total, except for carrots, beets and other sweet starchy vegetables listed on page 221.

There is no limit on green vegetable intake.

This is a good place to mention fat. Fat does not make you fat. Starch and sugar taken to excess will. Lets take a look at why fat is useful for you and the kind of fats to choose.

Adequate fat can affect hormone function as well as calm down a fragile nervous system. Look at the numbers of people that take fat out of the diet. They can be tired, pale, edgy, have poor skin tone, become forgetful or suffer from irregular if not missed periods and other hormone related issues — why? A major hormone precursor is cholesterol. Lowering fats can affect cholesterol levels thus contributing to hormone imbalances.

Choose a fat that has not been altered by the addition of chemicals to lengthen shelf life, heated to keep the fat from spoiling or changed from a natural vegetable oil form to create a margarine or spread.

Imagine being able to eat real butter — that's right 2-4 teaspoons of butter a day would actually be good for you. No more it's barely butter, if your eyes are half closed it's butter, if you stand on your head it's butter — go get the butter!

I recommend olive oil, butter, nut and seed oils such as sesame, flax walnut, coconut oil or almond oils and as well as fish oil — cod liver oil, halibut oil or salmon oil. These are unprocessed, healthy oils and contain many valuable nutrients.

Chapter 9

An Easy-to-Follow
Low-Carbohydrate Plan

For the first two weeks, here is an easy guideline to follow. I consider it a little rigid but it can be a useful kick-start to following a low-carbohydrate plan.

For the first two weeks, plan to keep your carbohydrate gram intake at approximately 30 grams per day. At the end of two weeks on 30 grams per day program, I suggest that you increase your daily carbohydrate gram intake to 60 grams per day and expand your food horizons at this time.

You can eat any amount of meat, fish, poultry and eggs (providing you have no sensitivities to these items) and vegetables at each meal. Butter, nuts, and oils may also be consumed in limited amounts. If you are overweight, you probably will have allergies or sensitivities to dairy products, cheese, milk and cream.

Choose green vegetables, as they are low in carbohydrates.

Keep your intake of starchy vegetables low. For example: 1 cup cooked winter squash = 10 grams of carbohydrate, and 1 medium sized sweet potato = 20 grams of carbohydrate.

Vegetable Choices

Eat any amount of the following vegetables, cooked or raw.

Arugula, asparagus, bean sprouts, bok choy, broccoli, cabbage, cauliflower, celery, collard greens, crookneck squash, cucumber, endive, escarole, fresh herbs, green pepper, kale, kohlrabi, lettuce, patti-pan squash, parsley, radishes, spinach, su choy, summer squash, watercress, zucchini.

Starchy Vegetable Choices

For the first two weeks of your program, keep your consumption of these vegetables low. (Refer to a complete list of carbohydrates for verification.)

Artichokes, avocado, beets, Brussels sprouts, butternut squash, carrots, Danish squash, eggplant, jicama, leeks, okra, olives, onion, pumpkin, sweet potatoes, tomatoes, turnips, water chestnuts, winter squash, yams.

Beverages

Herbal or decaffeinated teas or coffee, coffee substitutes, beef or chicken broth, and lots of purified water. Stay away from alcohol despite what other diet books say.

Fruits

Consume fresh fruits on a limited basis as snacks only and watch carbohydrate grams. Usually ½ to 1 piece of fresh fruit per day.

Here is a surprising look at some carbohydrate grams.

1 slice bread = 20–25 grams
1 medium potato = 20 grams
1 cup cooked rice = 20 grams
1 ear of corn = 20 grams
2 Ry Krisp (100% whole rye) crackers = 14 grams
1 rice cake = 8–13 grams
15 almonds or 1/4 cup = 5 grams
1/2 avocado = 5 grams

Refer to carbohydrate gram chart on page 217 or to low-carbohydrate diet books for a complete list of foods and information.

Next we will discuss the fourth important component of successful weight loss — exercise — not excessive, but daily.

Chapter 10

Exercise

Yes it's time to address exercise but now it's going to be easy. This time, you won't be caring around all those toxins that are making you feel tired and sluggish. You'll be clear and your energy and the natural desire to move and exercise will return. Exercise is an important component of any weight loss or health program. Don't despair the dreaded *E* word can really be pleasant. When the word exercise is mentioned, most people conjure up an image of hours of sweating it out in the gym, or being terrified to go to the gym because they feel so out of shape. Fortunately there are many programs and classes that cater to overweight people.

When I am with a client, I will get a sense of the amount of exercise that they are currently doing. For a high energy type, a slow, steady, rhythmic exercise such as tai chi, yoga or swimming might be more beneficial than what they are currently doing, which might be nothing or something too strenuous. These people can be calmed through the action of slow, focused exercise incorporating specific movements, which require being in the present moment. Heavier, more sedentary types would probably respond to something more energetic like boxing, Tae-Bo, weightlifting, fast walking or running.

Most of the time, I sense that more intense exercise on a cardio-vascular level seems to be required. In the case of overweight or out-of-shape people, I usually hear a loud groan when cardiovascular exercise is mentioned and the thought of a sweaty body pounding it out on the pavement brings terror to their hearts. None of this is necessary. The body just wants you to move.

Ask yourself what type of exercise would be beneficial for your body and make the commitment to do it every day.

I like cross country skiing in the winter and swimming in the summer. If I don't exercise for a few days if I am traveling and I am away from my routine, I just don't feel like myself. I am healthy and full of energy so my body just naturally wants to move. This will be the case for you. The body will literally propel you out the door. You will have very little choice in the matter. What used to be a chore will become a pleasure.

Take a look at this letter from one of my clients:

Dear Caroline,

I didn't believe you when you said that my body would just feel like exercising. I didn't start to exercise right away. I waited until I had the response from my body. It took about two weeks. After following your Body Knows *food plan, I could feel my body just naturally wanting to move. I was ready for it. I treated myself to a new set of exercise shoes which I laced up and started out. There are a number of hills where I live. I set a goal to try and climb one of these hills. It was tough at first – a lot of huffing and puffing but now I can do it. Walking through my neighborhood has given me a greater sense of connection to the wonder of life and nature. I observe the trees and bushes — the plants coming into bloom, who is renovating their house and the stages of the renovation. I am able to appreciate all that I have so much more now that I am getting out and moving. I am still a plus size but my pants are now loose. I am not sure when I will feel like exercising with other people but for now I am happy and grateful for the steps I am taking and this new addition to my life.*

Your body knows the type of exercise that would be right for you. As soon as the energy just naturally courses into your body, which it will — then you move and let the universe guide you to explore many exercise options. Because the instincts of your body are directly linked to what will give you the most joy and the best form of exercise, something unexpected might be revealed. It could be tap dancing, swimming, Pilates, or ballet, as well as any traditional form of exercise.

I suggest to people that they lace up their athletic shoes and walk every day.

I suggest to people that they lace up their athletic shoes and walk every day.

Walk for about fifteen minutes and feel gratitude in your heart while you do it.

Every so often during your walk, put on a "head of steam" — power walk or walk like a duck for about 20–30 paces. Pick a marker — perhaps a tree or a telephone pole — power walk to that marker. Swing your arms, quicken your pace, and increase your heart rate. Just travel as far as you are comfortable. Every few days add another segment of power walking to your daily walk. In a few weeks you might even feel like a comfortable jog during one of these segments. The idea is to get the heart rate up, improve the function of the lymphatic system and increase those "feel good" brain chemicals into the body, which curb hunger pangs and improve attitude.

Many of my clients are overweight, but I remember Gavin in particular. His life long battle with the dieting game led him to me weighing over 200 pounds. When we discussed the importance of exercise he balked — there was just no way in his mind that he could do it. Although it was a tough commitment, somehow something I said about exercise rang true and he was motivated to put on his exercise shoes every day and walk. At first it was minimal — just around the block; then it increased to two blocks. Within a few weeks he had lost 15 pounds and could walk almost a mile. Gavin knew that in order to get that exercise component into his daily routine, he had to take that walk first thing in the morning. Then he was done for the day and feeling proud of his accomplishment. Exercise is a huge component in weight loss, and physical and mental well-being.

If you have exercise equipment, use your treadmill or exercise bike for five minutes a day for one or two weeks, then increase to five minutes twice daily. The body knows what you are doing and it will respond. Resist the temptation in the beginning to think that you have to exercise long and hard. Just do something.

I often recommend the use of a re-bounder or mini-trampoline, which can be a fun, cardiovascular exercise as well as less taxing to muscles and joints. It seems in this weightless state, as the body jumps, there may also be benefits to the lymphatic system.

Use the re-bounder for three minutes per day for the first ten days and then increase to three minutes twice a day and build up.

Now that we have discussed exercise, we are ready to shed light on the most important component of weight loss — hormones.

Chapter 11

Hormones

The last and most important component of successful weight loss is hormone balance — usually missing or rarely discussed in any popular diet book. If those hormones are not balanced, then you will not lose weight or you might lose weight initially and then plateau.

The last and most important component of successful weight loss is hormone balance — usually missing or rarely discussed in any popular diet book.

When I look into a physical body, I see the body in terms of the systems that are out of balance. One of the most common imbalanced systems is the endocrine system. Overweight people almost always have hormone imbalances.

All too often, people can blame themselves, their emotional issues, and past experiences when in my opinion, much of their mental anguish can stem from endocrine imbalances.

In terms of weight gain, hormone imbalances can contribute to overeating and that "never satisfied feeling."

In my own life as a menopausal woman, I know that my emotional well-being and maintaining my ideal weight has been greatly enhanced by the addition of bio-identical hormone balancing.

Let me tell you about Mary, who attended one of my weight-loss seminars. She had the usual problems associated with weight gain: Gas, bloating, fatigue, and overwhelming sugar cravings. She was also very emotional and frequently on the verge of tears. She had been everywhere seeking help not only for her weight problem, but with her constant weeping — to no avail.

When I met her, I "knew" right away that this was an endocrine problem, not an emotional one. Fortunately, I knew of a medical doctor in the city who specialized in bio-identical hormone balancing. I felt this would be useful. Through blood work and pinpointing the exact area of imbalance and providing the specific remedy to treat it, this woman was able to find relief at last.

Most people think that their hormones are located

in their pelvis but actually the master endocrine glands are actually located in the head!

> *Most people think that their hormones are located in their pelvis but the master endocrine glands are actually located in the head!*

For instance, the hypothalamus is an important endocrine gland that governs appetite, emotion, memory and hormone balance. The pineal gland responds to light and endocrine balance and the pituitary gland relates to growth. The thyroid gland located in the base of the neck regulates mood, temperature and weight control as well as effecting elimination! Many people may be suffering from what is known as sub-clinical low thyroid.

The Candida yeast syndrome, which I have discussed at length in these pages, can often contribute to a low functioning thyroid. The thyroid gland at the base of the neck is involved in maintaining body weight, fat metabolism, body temperature, energy and well-being. It is very often out of balance. Some doctors say that it is in epidemic proportions in this country. A medical test may not always detect a low thyroid. People with low thyroid will often have difficulty losing weight.

The use of certain herbs, botanicals, glandular materials, or synthetic thyroid medication will help this important gland to function correctly. For many people, it is as if the lights go on and the after-burners for energy and weight loss go up after the thyroid is balanced.

Here is a simple test to determine a possible subclinical low thyroid. This test is not scientific but may be an indication that your thyroid is not functioning optimally.

(Please note that liquid iodine can stain your clothes. Wear an old T-shirt)

- Purchase a bottle of liquid iodine at the health food store.
- Paint a 3 **x** 4 inch square patch on the inside of your upper arm. Roll up your T-shirt.
- Note that the color of the patch will be bright orange at first.
- Watch the patch over the next few hours and see if the bright color diminishes and fades. If the color fades rapidly, it could mean that your thyroid is soaking up the iodine, a useful element in thyroid regulation. It could be time to seek help from a skilled professional who will test you to determine if this is the case.

Insulin is another important hormone. Insulin, secreted by the pancreas, is responsible for blood sugar regulation. Lowering carbohydrates can help balance insulin levels thus contributing to improved hormone function. Cholesterol is another important component in the hormone balance equation. Many people with the best of intentions greatly reduce fats in the diet often affecting vital hormone function.

Many people with the best of intentions greatly reduce fats in the diet often effecting vital hormone function.

Men and women also suffer from low testosterone levels. Again, appropriate hormone balance will assist men and women (we all produce testosterone) in regaining energy, well-being and libido. Seek help from a physician or well-respected practitioner in your community with bio-identical or natural hormone balancing.

Stress can affect hormones. Constant stress and low blood sugar (hypoglycemia) can affect the stress hormones — adrenaline and cortisol.

Too much cortisol from stress and too much insulin in the blood affect adrenal function creating fatigue, irritability and weight gain. High cortisol levels can create excess weight around the waist and low cortisol levels could mean that it is impossible for the person to lose that weight. This can contribute to adrenal exhaustion. Call your local compounding pharmacy and ask for a list of medical doctors for whom they fill prescriptions, then call the doctors and choose one you feel comfortable working with.

If a person is trying to lose weight and they are following all of the appropriate guidelines of food allergies, limiting carbohydrate grams, exercising daily etc., and they have reached a plateau in their quest for the ideal body weight, it usually points to a hormone imbalance. It takes a person with a great deal more knowledge than I have in this regard to assist them. However, there are naturally based supplements as well as prescription medications available, which can help. When it comes to hormones and weight gain, don't blame yourself for attitudes and emotional states, seek help from a competent allopathic or holistic practitioner.

Emotions and Weight Gain

Many people who have weight problems may be coping with patterns of addiction or low self-esteem in the equation. An addiction is anything which has a *hold* on us such as: overwork, exercise, sex, food, chocolate, sugar, coffee, alcohol, cigarettes, illegal drugs, medications, money, worry, material possessions, relationships, negativity, over achieving, gambling etc. People can also be addicted to illness.

The grapple hook of addictions can be an avoidance mechanism to take us off the path to fulfillment or to prevent us from exploring issues and subjects that expose our vulnerability.

These addictive tendencies begin in childhood and our constant need for attention. Some people have had very traumatic childhoods. The comfort that their addiction provides is justifiable.

Our parents or caregivers kept us quiet with food, the breast, the pacifier, the bottle, the toys, the outings, the diversions — and the minute we squawked, we were given something to keep us quiet. As adults, we rely upon these addictions to numb the pain and frustration of daily life. These items give us a sense of power and control.

Coffee drinkers, for example, can describe in minute detail the feeling of their special brand of elixir as it touches every inch of their alimentary tract. And yet, you wouldn't believe the numbers of people who are seeking optimum health while being addicted to caffeine, chocolate and sugars, not to mention illegal drugs, cigarettes, and alcohol. As soon as people stop taking these addictive substances, their health dramatically improves.

I believe that life is all about learning, growing, and mastering certain behaviors, the least of which are addictions. An addiction carries a negative force, a powerful force that is sapping our life force or vitality

When we implement the five components of weight loss in "The Body Knows Diet" program, and because we are satisfied with non-allergic foods and calmed or inspired by our new program and the way we feel, this helps us to overcome additions to unhealthy foods and behaviors.

From the spiritual perspective, nothing must have a

hold over us — no substance, person, place or possession. On a spiritual level, we must be free, clear, and available to be moved by the universe. The addictions derail us and keep us from fully entering life and our true calling. Staying stuck in an addiction to any behavior means that we are not really ready to grow up and take full responsibility for the life that God has given us.

> *Staying stuck in an addiction to any behavior means that we are not really ready to grow up and take full responsibility for the life that God has given us.*

In another way, if we are addicted, we are not clear. We do not radiate clear, positive energy to others around us. We appear listless, dull, tired and worn down.

We desire to manifest the best into our lives on a material and spiritual level. I believe that the emanation of this radiant, positive energy, which comes from having a clear and healthy physical body, and plenty of personal fulfillment through our work and our relationships, is the cornerstone to bringing positive experiences into our lives.

On an emotional level, an addicted person has a very strong little girl or boy inside them who is running the show.

> *On an emotional level, an addicted person*
> *has a very strong little girl or boy inside*
> *them who is running the show.*

"Life is too difficult and I must have my treats, my pacifier, or something to make me feel better," we say.

Here is an interesting account of one woman's struggle with addictions:

I am a woman who has struggled with my weight since I was 10 years old and, like so many stories you've read, I have tried all the "diets" over the years. But, trust me, the Body Knows Diet is different!

I am in my 50s, overweight and making excuses for why I feel sluggish, why my knees hurt, why my legs are tired, and why my feet hurt. I told myself it was because of my weight, my age and lack of exercise – so it was to be expected.

I'd known about Caroline's program for seven years, but was unwilling to commit. You know what I mean – all of you who want to do something but it just seems too hard.

Well…. I finally reached that desperation point last October. I gave up the sugar, wheat, etc. I started losing 10–15–20 lbs. I was feeling more energetic, walking with a little spring in my step, and my incentive was the loss of weight.

By Christmas I had lost 31 lbs. I was so thrilled and I decided to reward myself. I told myself as a special treat I could eat whatever I wanted for Christmas day. Dressing, potatoes, pie, fudge — I had it all.

Well, you guessed it: Three months later I was still "rewarding" myself. Like any addiction, as soon as I started it got out of control again. But that's not the news!

Three weeks — just three weeks *after I started eating sugar again I had an epiphany! I got out of bed one morning and limped to the bathroom, suddenly realizing that* I hadn't been limping and there hadn't been any pain!

If you remember nothing else, remember this! It took just three weeks of eating poorly, of giving in to my addiction to sweets for the pain to return. I had been feeling so good that I didn't even realize the pain was gone and now it was back.

Needless to say, I have the incentive and the determination once again and all I have to do is stay on The Body Knows Diet program for a world of difference in my life.

I know for sure that what we eat does make a difference, and knowing our food allergies can make a difference in pain, symptoms, and effective weight loss. I am so thankful to Caroline.

When people realize that the body they have been given is an instrument to carry them through their destiny and purpose in this life, then people seem happy to let go of the addictions in favor of a healthier lifestyle.

I'm often asked how I manage my own food cravings. Like many of you, I have a strong *inner child* that needs plenty of nurturing. I have to let the little child have her treats — treats which will not make me feel sick. Because I am very aware of my food sensitivities, I had to do a lot of research and tweaking of recipes to find goodies that would not make my Candida proliferate, not spike my blood sugar (which would give me that tired, low energy feeling later on), and not initiate a histamine reaction which would trigger food allergies and consequent weight gain from fluid retention.

On occasion, I do enjoy a sweet dessert or a glass of wine. I indulge myself occasionally, but it has to be something really special. For instance, I might be willing to pay the price for feeling a little "off" the next day for a delectable slice of hazelnut torte or a dish of crème brulée. But it is not worth it for me to jeopardize my program for a mundane piece of pie or just an ordinary cookie.

When, like me, you know your body so well that you can tell when it is slightly left of center, the foods that you used to crave will not have a hold on you. The value that you will place on a finely tuned, healthy body will be too great.

Chapter 13

Getting Started
on Your Program

While I write this book I am thinking of each one of you and wanting every success from this "Body Knows Diet" program for you and for everyone who is tired of the weight loss game.

I know the five components of weight loss intimately and have taught this program to thousands of people. I have been very successful for the past 20 years in assisting people to lose weight and I am gratified by their many testimonials and stories. I know what it feels like to be overweight, tired and sluggish and I know how good it feels to have maintained my ideal weight and to have mental clarity and boundless energy. This is your birthright too! Find a friend and team up.

Now it is time to take the first step. You must believe first of all that you are worth it and second of all that it will be easy and that you can do it — and you can!

Get ready!

Use the following affirmations and motivating points to get started and stay the course with your weight loss program. Copy and cut out the affirmations, then tape them to your refrigerator or bathroom mirror. Always remember to check with your doctor before starting any new program.

I am ready to lose weight. Because I now understand the five components of weight-loss, I can be successful.

I clean out my cupboards and refrigerator of all foods which contain sugar, caffeine, chemicals and allergy-containing foods. I read labels.

I team up with a friend who communicates to me every day about my diet plan and food choices. We motivate each other to stay on track with our "Body Knows Diet" program.

When I slip up, my friend is there to bring me back to center and to my deep desire to stay on my program. I motivate her and she/he motivates me. We do not give up on each other. If we inadvertently cheat, we do not completely de-rail but re-focus and get back on track immediately.

I love my body and am excited about the new changes.

Every day I lace up my exercise shoes and go for a walk, go to the gym or swim. Or I use my in-home exercise equipment. I make time early in the morning before my day begins. I love my exercise routine. My body loves to exercise.

I shop wisely, plan ahead and cook nourishing and satisfying meals. I follow "The Body Knows Diet Food Plan" (on page 191) and enjoy preparing the low carbohydrate, allergy-free recipes in "The Body Knows" cookbook.

I snack on protein, veggies, nuts or seeds and resist the temptation to get back into sweets or carbs. If I need a "pretend cookie," I take cashew nut butter or almond butter and spread it on a 100% rye or rice cracker. Yum!

I see that I am losing weight. I choose not to look at the scales but to observe how my clothes are fitting and how good and clear my skin looks.

I have been on my program for _____ weeks. I am pleased with my progress.

I re-script my mind with my "Why Wait to Lose Weight" CD, which I play as I fall asleep at night. The program helps me to relax and reassures me that my body is able to lose weight easily and effortlessly. I feel peaceful and joyful as my body responds to the new changes.

I seek help in balancing my hormones through my medical doctor, pharmacist or holistic practitioner.

Chapter 14

Typical Questions and Answers

Food-Related Questions

I never knew that food allergies or sensitivities could be at the root of my problem. How do I cut through the maze of exposures to these foods not only in my own kitchen but "out in the world" as well.

Choose foods other than "the big five" — that's all! Eat heartily from the "non offending" food list. See "*The Body Knows Diet* Food Plan" on page 191. Enjoy the delicious recipes in *The Body "Knows" Cookbook*.

How am I going to manage without wheat and bread? Wheat or flour are everywhere!

Substitute rice, potatoes, 100% rye bread, rice bread, rye crackers, rice cakes, rice crackers, sweet potatoes, yams, squash or unusual grains such as millet, amaranth, quinoa and buckwheat. Guess what — you'll lose weight because you are not triggering histamine reactions. Be careful of corn — a common allergen and very sweet. And you *must* count carbohydrate grams. Check the gram counter on page 217.

You may not be triggering a histamine reaction, in your food choices but remember that you may be consuming too many carbohydrates. Stick to approximately 60 grams on a permanent on-going basis.

Avoid wheat to the best of your ability for thirty days — or longer if necessary. Remember that wheat is wheat is wheat. White bread, brown bread, sprouted wheat, low-carb wheat bread or low-calorie wheat crackers — any kind of wheat flour in any form should be eliminated. I have also seen wheat-allergic people react to wheat grass and to cosmetics containing wheat germ.

Now that you're not initiating a histamine reaction from wheat and flour based products, you'll lose weight as stored fluid is released from the tissue. It can happen within the first two days. But remember that you have to avoid *all* "the big five" foods from your diet at once. For instance, you may eliminate wheat but you may be allergic to soy so that needs to be eliminated as well, in order for your program to be successful.

For years, I have enjoyed a bag of popcorn as a late night snack. Popcorn is recommended in so many diet books as being a beneficial low-calorie choice. Now you are saying that I could be allergic to corn — why?

Corn is among the five common allergic foods. Not only are you consuming popcorn every day but corn is widely used in the baking industry because it is a sweet (high fructose corn syrup) and cheap filler. Corn is found in many packaged foods — even toothpaste! Corn is high in carbohydrate — an ear of corn contains 23 grams of carbohydrate — almost half your daily allotment of 60 grams.

Despite what all the diet books say, I do not recommend that people go to bed hungry. If you are hungry — eat!

Choose a protein based snack before going to bed. *Do not overeat.* Celery sticks stuffed with almond or cashew nut butter, a hard-boiled egg or cold chicken leg will settle down your pancreas, not cause a fluctuation in blood sugar and will help you to sleep whereas a bag of popcorn quickly turns to sugar, which converts to fat while you sleep. Then in the morning, you are likely to be wearing that bag of popcorn around your waist!

You talk about 30 days — why is a 30 day program so important?

It takes a few days for histamine reactions to subside. The effect of a histamine reaction from food allergies can remain in the body for upwards of 48 hours. Fluid starts to be released from the body — usually after 12 hours. Then the body starts to adjust to the new program. As toxins are eliminated and allergic reactions diminish, a sense of well being returns to the body. Often pain or inflammatory reactions subside as well. Then the person starts to experience a sense of well-being with increased energy and vitality. This is the crucial time. This is not the time to get back into offending foods but to stay the course and keep going for another few weeks until new eating patterns are well established.

I find that staying away from social settings or restaurant temptations really helps at least for the first 14 days of your "Body Knows Diet" program. A 30-day program will show you what the body can do for you. Thirty days is just a start: This is really an ongoing, permanent program.

How can I expect to feel after being on my program for 30 days?

Usually you will experience a noticeable improvement in your energy, mental clarity and a change in your waistline. Most of the complaints you had 30 days ago will be greatly diminished. If you are disciplined, you will be able to eat the occasional offending food. You may enjoy a sweet dessert, a glass of wine, an exposure to dairy products, or another "no-no" food very occasionally and your body will probably say, "Fine,

I can handle that!" Over exposure to offending foods may cause your symptoms and excess pounds to return. Many people on my weight-loss program choose to be on a very strict program with no "sins" and no cheating for 60 days. By then a good routine has been established and they are not as likely to be tempted by sweets, wine or offending foods.

I have heard about food "rotation" what does that mean?

After your 30-day avoidance program and the establishment of your new eating program, you may introduce wheat or an offending food on an occasional basis, such as once every fifth day. This process is called *rotation*, a procedure that avoids the overexposure of a food or substance and prevents the body from becoming allergic or sensitive to that substance due to multiple exposures. People become sensitive to foods that they consume every single day. *But be careful even of rotation.*

If you have addictive tendencies and more than 20 pounds to lose, avoid wheat and flour-based products as well as all the other big five items for as long as you can and *never* bring them home to your own kitchen.

I understand that wheat/flour, barley and oats are related – please explain?

While you are avoiding wheat, it can be helpful to avoid oats and barley for the first 30 days, because these too are *glutinous grains*. After 30 days these may be re-introduced. But remember oats and barley are high in carbohydrate.

I suggest that 100% whole rye, in the form of delicious breads or crackers, can be tolerated because of its low-gluten content. One hundred percent rye bread is delicious toasted or as a base for open-faced sandwiches for lunch. But remember even one slice of 100% rye bread will contain approximately 25 grams of carbohydrate. I prefer 100% rye crackers, which contain less carbohydrate.

Why is fruit a problem? I thought we were supposed to eat five servings of fruits per day.

Fruit is sugar. Too much sugar converts to fat in the system. Fruit, fruit juice, dried fruit are all sugars and may contribute to blood sugar handling problems, hypoglycemia, an overtaxed pancreas, and feed yeast. Keep sugars very low and keep fruits to a minimum — ½ to 1 piece a day. Choose fruits that are lower in carbohydrate grams. One cup of watermelon contains approximately 11 grams of carbohydrate. A small bowl of raspberries is 8 grams. A mango for example contains 20 and a banana 25. Fruits do contain nutrients and fiber but there may be downside to consuming too many.

I bless everyone who attends my workshops. But I see thousands of people who can be quite out of balance and even emotionally unstable because they think they are doing themselves a favor by consuming large quantities of fruit! These well-intentioned people can be hypoglycemic or borderline diabetic.

The solution is to increase your vegetable intake — eat lots of green leafy vegetables and keep your fruit consumption low.

I always thought that honey is healthy. Why is it off the list?

Honey is a sugar. Sugar feeds yeast. There are 15 grams of carbohydrate in 1 tablespoon of honey.

I get constipated every time I follow a low-carbohydrate program. Why is that? And do you have any suggestions for chronic constipation?

You've read my story: How I was constipated for years because of food allergies. Once you stop consuming offending foods, bowel movements usually became regular. Also, Candida albicans yeast affects gut flora balance. I suggest taking some lactobacillus acidophilus capsules on a daily basis, drink lots of water, increase fibrous vegetables. Try taking about 250 mg. of magnesium at bedtime. If that doesn't do it, take a look at your thyroid. Low thyroid function can often result in constipation.

I have been on a low-carbohydrate program and have consumed copious amounts of cheese and other dairy products. How am I going to manage without these dairy products?

Dairy products are much easier to avoid than wheat products. Dairy products are always a choice. You are either pouring the milk, cutting the cheese, or spooning out the ice cream.

Goat's milk and goat's milk cheese and sheep's cheese may be tolerated because they are a different food family. (Refer to food families on page 221.) Some people may experience symptoms, such as weight gain or nasal congestion from drinking cow's milk but cheese, yogurt or cultured cow's milk products may be tolerated. Wait 30 days before trying *any* dairy product — even sheep and goat products. Then introduce them and note any reactions notably to sinus symptoms or weight gain from fluid retention.

The body knows, and your symptoms will tell you.

In response to your question, I suggest that you use nuts and seeds or small amounts of protein for snacks. You may need some form of calcium supplementation if you are avoiding dairy products

Will I ever be able to eat wheat or dairy products again?

Of course, as long as you remember not to ingest the offending items frequently — no more than every fifth day, on a rotation basis, covered in an earlier question. But watch for weight gain from fluid retention — one of the biggest signs of a dairy or wheat allergy. Here's how I do it. I never bring cow's milk dairy products into my own kitchen. Occasionally especially during the summer, I have sheep or goats milk cheese. The reason why I am more able to tolerate these products during the summer is that there are less environmental molds in the air at that time of year. Cheese contains mold. Molds are a common allergen.

How can I live without coffee?

When it comes to making healthy changes, probably, my most commonly asked question is, "How can I replace coffee — or black tea?

Quite simply, the very best way you can — as soon as you can, with something that won't derail your nervous system, over-stimulate your adrenal glands, agitate your pancreas, increase your heart rate, dull your complexion, clog your liver or give you urinary problems.

Caffeine stimulates a temporary surge in blood sugar, which can be followed by an over-production of insulin and consequent low-blood sugar downward spiral.

Delicious herbal teas are readily available, decaffeinated coffee and tea may be taken in very limited amounts, and remember to drink 6–8 glasses of water a day.

I have a very stressful job and I look forward to a relaxing glass of wine when I get home from work. If wine is off the list what am I to do?

In my opinion, relaxing as alcohol might be, you may be setting yourself up for an unhealthy addiction if you consume it every night. I suggest a run, walk or a meditation might be a better way to unwind. However, a non-fermented low-carbohydrate distilled liquor like gin or vodka might be a better choice than wine, which contains more carbohydrate plus the chemicals and ferments that can feed yeast or trigger an allergic reaction.

Mix ½ oz. with soda, a squeeze of lime, a drop or two of stevia and some ice, you have a refreshing drink. Less alcohol still gives you the "buzz" but not the downside the next morning.

Is there a downside to implementing these dietary changes?

You could experience "withdrawal" symptoms for a few days. This is a natural detoxification reaction. This is when the body is releasing toxins into the blood stream and you could experience symptom exacerbation, low energy or feel a little achy. Drink plenty of water, take some vitamin C, get to bed early and "ride it out." Some people experience none of these symptoms but occasionally a few will. But the upside is that in a few days you will feel better, less symptomatic, more energetic and have more mental clarity — all worth the few days of detox and release of all those poisons you've been putting into your system for so many years!

Why would food allergies be such an issue in our culture? Don't people in other countries have these problems too?

The American diet is largely responsible for food allergies. Multiple exposures to common foods, heavy dependence on packaged and processed foods and overeating puts stress on our stomachs and digestive systems. Other cultures don't overeat the way we do, food is fresh and less processed and varies from season to season. However, I do see people from other cultures with food allergies — notably to dairy products and wheat products which become apparent when they arrive in this country, adopt our eating habits and develop allergies.

Will I ever be clear of these allergies?

Yes, when you relieve your body of stress and work consistently on your emotional issues. In the meantime, a period of avoidance is the most practical solution in order to relieve pressure from the immune system, reduce histamine reactions and release stored fluid from your body.

You might consider investigating acupuncture,

homeopathy, a cleansing program, allergy desensitizing techniques, or other forms of treatment offered through an alternative medical clinic for relief.

(For more in-depth information regarding the day-to-day management of food allergies, refer to *"The Body Knows Diet* Food Plan" on page 191. This basic plan, which usually works well for most people, will round out your knowledge and answer more of your questions. It will also give you tips for snacks, traveling, and dining out.)

There's a lot of talk about food combining. I try to do it right, but I keep forgetting not to combine my proteins and starches. Is there another solution?

Successful food combining means consuming proteins and vegetables together at one meal, and starches and vegetables together at another, with a two-hour break between. Fruit should be consumed by itself, two hours before or two hours after a meal. Whew — this can get a little confusing!

Simplify things and enjoy a little food freedom: Take digestive enzymes with each meal. Many varieties are available at the health-food store. Enzymes help the body to break down and absorb food — plus they cut down gas and bloating.

Candida-Related Questions

What about alcohol?

Ideally, if you are eradicating Candida albicans, then wine and beer need to be avoided, because they are fermented beverages that also contain yeasts. Yeast, molds and ferments can trigger reactions — and carbohydrate grams in alcohol mount up.

But hard liquor, such as vodka or scotch may be allowed because it is distilled and not fermented and is lower in carbohydrate than wine or beer. The occasional ounce *may* be permissible — but not for the first 30 days until your healthy eating habits are established. Stick to mineral water with a squeeze of lime.

You will notice that as you avoid excessive carbohydrates, sweets, starches and alcohol that your energy and sense of well-being dramatically shifts — you feel fabulous.

You will notice that as you avoid excessive carbohydrates, sweets, starches and alcohol that your energy and sense of well-being dramatically shifts — you feel fabulous.

This is the way you are supposed to feel. Alcohol, more than a few sips, elevates insulin levels and creates a blood sugar imbalance, diminishing that wonderful feeling.

If you are working on a Candida yeast eradication program, any sort of fermented food should be avoided such as: cheese, mushrooms, soy sauce, pickles, and vinegar.

Headaches or post-nasal drip are common symptoms associated with yeast or mold sensitivity.

I have had a weight problem for 30 years. I am afraid that I may derail after following my 30 day program and get back into my old habits. What do you suggest?

Keep a watchful eye on the Candida yeast syndrome. Remember this is one of the key reasons *why* you have had cravings — probably for decades.

This is the biggest place where people get derailed. After about 21–30 days on your program, you will notice that you no longer have cravings for starches and sugars or they are much less and under control. Stay the course.

As soon as you get a craving, look immediately for a protein snack. A small amount of protein will settle down a craving and "hold you" until you are able to sit down to a regular meal.

My advice is to keep offending foods out of your own kitchen. Don't bring them home and then, after 30 days, if you are tempted, enjoy an occasional treat away from home, but get right back on track with your low-carbohydrate, allergy free program. If you continue to consume starches and sugars again — those old familiar cravings will return with a vengeance and you will feel bloated, tired and groggy to boot!

Often, I notice that when people get off track, they are overcome by cravings for starches and sugars and the cycle repeats itself.

Continue to work on Candida with your anti-candida supplementation and take it on a daily basis. This is usually the area where people get into trouble and forget the importance of diligence in Candida eradication.

Because of Candida, I'm avoiding sugars and juice. What do I do for sweets?

Usually a person who craves starches and sugars needs more or consistent protein. Try choosing protein for a snack. The protein will "hold" you longer.

For a sweet snack, try a rice cracker with some almond or cashew nut butter and a tiny sprinkle of Stevia (a natural herbal sweetener) on it. Stevia is available in powder or liquid form at the health food store.

There are other alternative sweeteners such as Aspartame, Xylitol, Splenda® or Sucralose® (an altered sugar, used in diet foods and low-carbohydrate snacks) that are available in grocery and health food stores. But these sugar substitutes are synthesized or man-made and research has shown that there may be some concern about the safe long-term use of these items. Stevia is a safe natural sweetener.

Nutrasweet® is a synthesized sweetener made from an amino-acid combination. Splenda is an altered sugar substance and is widely used in diet foods and soft drinks. I have met with clients who have consumed and been addicted to these diet drinks and they tell me that when they stop consuming them that life-long symptoms have subsided.

Nutrasweet®, or aspartame, has received much negative press. Personally, when I chew gum containing this substance I notice that my throat feels dry. That is an indication of a mild allergic reaction.

I remember one client, who consumed three large bottles of diet soda per day and who suffered from emotional upheavals and severe anxiety. She calmed down and was able to discontinue medication when she stopped consuming diet drinks.

Trust your own instincts and take note of any symptoms or side effects when using anything but a natural sweetener.

I feel that sugar substitutes can be an important *temporary transition* away from excess cravings and sugar consumption. I discourage long-term use of anything that is not naturally derived. But just knowing that your cravings for sweets will diminish after your Candida yeast is under control is one of the positive side benefits and helps you to feel confident that in time, just a few short weeks, you will not even need a sugar substitute.

In just a few short weeks, you will not even need a sugar substitute.

Personally, I have no sugar cravings and it has nothing to do with will power. I have a box of powdered stevia in my kitchen which I rarely use. I don't have sugar cravings because:

- I eradicate Candida albicans yeast.
- I keep my sugars and starches low.
- My hormones are balanced

Hormone-Related Questions

I have been on a weight-loss program for three months and I have reached a plateau — what do I do now?

With every good intention, you may be exposing yourself to "offending foods" through your food choices — namely dairy products. Remember the big 5 food allergies — dairy, wheat, corn, soy and yeast not to mention sugar and caffeine. Eliminate all of these from the diet and usually the weight starts to drop again. If that doesn't help, then the glitch is hormones. Seek help from a local practitioner.

My daughter has been on birth control pills for the past year. I find her to be very moody and she constantly craves sweets.

Probably the most frustrating and complex issue that a woman of childbearing age has to face is the issue of birth control. Because so many women, whether they're married or not, are sexually active today, this can be a frequent, if not daily, dilemma.

Birth control pills are not always the answer for some women. Like any other medication, they are not for everyone. All too often, I see beautiful young women with the best of intentions suffering the negative effects of the birth control pill. Obviously, the pills are effective in preventing an unwanted pregnancy, but because they can alter a woman's delicate hormone balance, there are often unwanted side effects — namely Candida yeast.

I suggest that your daughter greatly reduce her intake of sweets, include protein at meals and snacks and seek help in Candida yeast eradication.

I am a 60 year-old post-menopausal woman. I was skinny as a rail up until 5 years ago. Now I have a noticeable roll around my tummy — it's demoralizing!

Menopause is a time when we have a tendency to put on weight and this can be so frustrating especially when many of us are not overeating!

During the pre (before), peri (in the middle of), or post (after) menopausal years, there are changes taking place in the body that we need to be aware of.

The endocrine system — which comprises the pineal, hypothalamus, pituitary, thyroid, parathyroid, adrenal glands, and reproductive organs — are changing and slowing down. Even though we may be missing body parts related to the reproductive system, the endocrine glands are still functioning, albeit not the way they were in our 30s and early 40s. We want to encourage the glands to function optimally as we continue to age. This can be accomplished with diet, nutritional supplements and hormone compounds both natural and synthesized. This is a delicate balance but with expert help, it can be achieved.

Weight gain, because of endocrine imbalances, tends to build up around the waist. This is called *omentum* — the extra band of fatty, estrogen-related tissue, which hangs like an apron around the middle. This excess adipose tissue is called estrogen dominance. Men are just as prone to this middle-age spread as women. We try to hide this stored fat by wearing oversized clothing, but by identifying food allergies and avoiding those offending foods as well as reducing carbohydrates, the omentum level can decrease. But the important quest at this time of your life is to balance hormones.

Weight gain in menopausal women can also be related to high estrogen levels. Soy has an estrogenic effect and can increase estrogen levels. It is a common allergen — one of the big five because of its indigestibility (it's a bean) and association with endocrine imbalances. Soy can suppress thyroid function and may block the absorption of iron and B vitamins. If you are overweight, you might want to decrease your soy intake.

What is the difference between natural and synthetic hormones?

Hormones that are chemically similar to those found in the human body are called natural or bio-identical. Plant-based or herbal formulas can be used to balance hormones. Synthetic hormones are manufactured with a chemical make-up that is not found in the human body but mimics some of the body's natural hormonal activity.

Where am I going to get help with individual hormone balancing?

A very important element of menopause is seeking perfect endocrine balance. What you seek is to feel good emotionally and physically — calm, stable, and balanced with a great sense of well-being, boundless energy, libido, and zest for life. This is not impossible. Fortunately, there are many medical doctors, practitioners, and experts whose life work and expertise lies in balancing hormones. Do not rest until you find someone who can assist you in this area. I have found *Natural Hormone Balance for Women: look younger, feel stronger and live life with exuberance by Uzzi Reiss, M.D.* (Simon and Schuster) to be a very useful reference regarding hormone fluctuations at this stage of life.

While Dr Reiss's book discusses all of the elements of hormone balance, and takes the confusion out of essential medical information, I still encourage you to seek help from an expert, either traditional or alternative, who can give you individual attention. There is no "one size fits all" where hormones are concerned.

In order to find a competent local practitioner, ask your pharmacist for the name of a "compounding pharmacy" in your city. Compounding pharmacies create bio-identical (like your own) hormone prescriptions for men and women based on your blood work or saliva testing provided to them by your physician. Then call the compounding pharmacy and ask for the name of the medical doctors or practitioners they work with. Then choose the recommended practitioner.

Reference:
Women's International Pharmacy
Custom Compounded Prescriptions for Men and Women
2 Marsh Court
Madison, WI 53718
608-221-7800
www.womensinternational.com
e-mail: info@womensinternational.com

The menopausal woman is constantly changing on an endocrine level. Because your cycles and symptoms are always changing, you will be working with your practitioner on a regular basis throughout your life to achieve this balance. Yes, hormones need to be balanced — even into our 80s!

It is unlikely that the same hormone substance will help you to find this balance from the peri- through the post-menopausal years. Hormones are constantly changing, and the compounds needed to balance them need to change and reflect our symptoms and our blood or saliva levels. Some hormone compounds cause side effects. Know what these side effects are. Don't settle for weight gain and feeling crummy. Keep researching and asking questions. I believe that the future for men and woman, in terms of anti-aging, vitality, sexual vigor and well-being lies specifically tailored hormone compounds, which are calibrated on an individual basis to match the changing endocrine system.

Exercise and Lifestyle-Related Questions

I have a lot of cellulite. I work out at the gym every day and drink lots of water. Is there an answer for this?

Another part of the excess-flesh equation is the dreaded *cellulite*. And we don't have to be menopausal to accumulate this lumpy material. Women (and men) of all ages are plagued with it. I find that most women who know their food allergies, particularly to dairy products and caffeine, have almost no accumulation of cellulite. That's the good news.

I just can't seem to get down to exercising. I start with great enthusiasm and then give up after a few days. What can I do to stay motivated?

I find the best time to exercise is first thing in the morning. I'm a morning person so I'm up with the birds and either swimming or taking an early morning walk before I do anything else. Exercise used to be a chore for me, but many years ago — when I implemented the five components of weight loss — exercise became an automatic activity. My body just naturally wanted to move. The choice seemed to come from within just as much as my own personal motivation that exercising was a good thing to do.

And so it will be for you.

Within a few days of starting your program and

your body begins to detoxify, letting go of all the accumulated poisons and toxins from years of consuming alcohol, sugar and caffeine, your energy will return and lacing up those exercise shoes will just be something that you "have to do."

My advice on exercise is: stick to something you love and can make a commitment to. For me there has to be a wonderful reward — a special treat — a gift in the activity.

I love to walk early in the morning. I love the smells and sounds of nature. I appreciate the season changes and feel blessed to have a healthy body with which to enjoy them. My walk becomes a meditation. I will often find a feather — a sign that "the angels are with me" or see a rainbow that affirms my belief in miracles.

Swimming is another early-morning pleasure. I swim in my pool before our Northwest summer begins. Then, I'm an ocean swimmer. There's nothing more therapeutic than a swim in the ocean — early in the morning and again before dinner. Salt water on the skin is nature's wonderful, healing body lotion.

I am originally from Austria, and in the European culture I have noticed that obesity is less prevalent than here in America — why is this?

Like you, I grew up in Europe. The one element that stands out is lifestyle. European people have a tremendous zest for life, an appreciation for humor, beauty, family, culture and history. Food for them is something to be savored, enjoyed, appreciated and shared.

A meal in France can span several hours. A meal in our culture can be "hoovered up" in a matter of minutes — sometimes seconds.

Food is a different concept and the pace especially at mealtimes more relaxed. In our country I feel that we are feeding the soul with food whereas in Europe the soul is fed through the richness of the culture, and food is only a part of it.

Shopping is different in Europe. People don't have access to the vast array of packaged foods that we do — nor the huge supermarkets. Use of chemicals, pesticides and additives is not as widespread. People shop on a daily basis and choose market available food.

Nor is the use of antibiotics in milk, meat and poultry production as prevalent thus Candida yeast, according to what health professionals in Europe tell me, is not in such epidemic proportions.

Women especially in France and Italy tend to be "chic" and well groomed. They are very interested in their bodies and want to keep them "mince" or trim. In France, for example, it is common practice to have a series of treatments, once a year for the "fois" — the liver. There are homeopathic pharmacies on almost every street corner and spas are a way of life — albeit for the people who can afford them.

Chapter 15

Clothes and Colors

When people are overweight there is a tendency to give up on one's appearance and let oneself go. I have been overweight. Believe me: black is the color of choice. We can hide away in the dark colors and the voluminous shirts. No one knows but us the secrets that our yards of cloth do not reveal.

Before I got involved in health education, I had a career in fashion. Black and any dark color is an excellent way to conceal extra pounds. But color — carefully chosen to match your skin, hair and eyes — can be magnetic. People can be drawn to you just by the colors you are wearing.

I suggest that you wear a bright and flattering color around the face while those pounds are coming off. Men can pair a bright (deep blue, purple, yellow or pink) shirt underneath a dark suit and the eye will be drawn to the face and not the waistline. Women can choose a bright shell or scarf under suit, dress or coat.

But just think: When you go on "The Body Knows Diet" program, your days for wearing dark garments will be numbered and color will be your friend again.

During your whole weight-loss program you want to look, feel, and be your best. The energy in your body will automatically make you feel this way. If you follow each of the five components of weight loss, you will see significant results.

The pay off will be purchasing some wonderful new clothes.

Research your most flattering clothing styles. Know which colors bring out your best features and help you to come alive. This is for your own well being. You are delivering a message every time you present yourself. You are making a statement and attracting people and experiences to you as a result of how you feel inside.

Stop at the cosmetic counter and get some suggestions on make up and the best colors to enhance your skin tone. Buy a new lipstick — a simple way to add color. Speak to your hair stylist about a cut, streaks or hair color.

You are coming out of the closet.

During my time as a fashion writer, we frequently gave women and men make-overs. As each person was made over from head to toe on the outside, with new clothes, make-up and hairstyles, the person changed on the inside: s/he invariably became more confident, outgoing, and happy as a result of the new look.

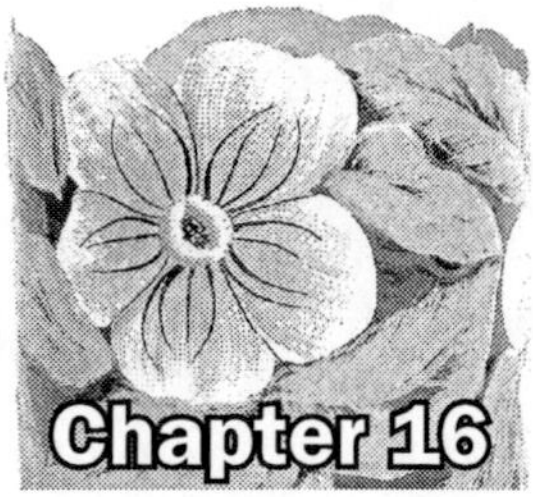

Chapter 16

The Benefits of Losing Weight

When we lose weight, we no longer shrink back and remain shadowed in obscurity. Because of the change in diet and balanced blood sugars and hormones, we have new-found energy and it is our time to shine. The benefits of weight loss are not just about feeling good.

I believe that everyone has special talents and a higher destiny or calling in this world, and when we lose weight our body chemistry changes and we are able to access the energy and mental clarity to be creative and productive.

It is natural during the weight-loss process, especially when we give up our addictions to common foods and beverages, that the body naturally detoxifies and releases stored chemicals and toxins. It doesn't take long before we feel more vital and energetic.

Not only that, but there are numerous health benefits:

the pancreas, the organ responsible for blood-sugar regulation, will be less taxed. You are no longer under the grapple hook of sugar addictions, so you are no longer tired or depressed. The liver is less burdened by toxins, the heart is less stimulated from allergic reactions, and the immune system is less over-loaded from the assault of environmental factors, common foods and assorted allergens. There are many benefits.

The biggest benefit is that YOU will emerge — the "you" that has been kept under wraps for a very long time. Watch out — get ready! Good things are going to happen.

When you follow your "Body Knows Diet" program, your energy and radiance will increase. You become magnetic. People will be attracted to you and your own natural energy will attract success, prosperity and an abundance of wonderful experiences. Here is a note from one of my clients outlining her experience.

"Caroline told me that I would become energetic and magnetic from her program. I started out, it took a few days and I began to feel different. The pounds just started to drop off. I had no idea how much water weight I was carrying. Within a week, I could see more clearly — I noticed the colors in the flowers and trees — something I had not noticed before. The colors seemed brighter and richer. I guess you could say I was more observant and more engaged in life —

more conscious and aware. It was as if I was waking up from a long dream. After a month people started noticing me and complimenting me. My whole attitude to life changed. It wasn't something I had to "try" to do — I just naturally felt better and happier. This is not a program it is a complete life change."

Chapter 17

Overweight Children

If you are concerned about your children or grand-children — their weight gain or obesity and their behavior problems, allergies, runny noses, crankiness, or poor energy — you will notice a dramatic difference when you eliminate sugar and dairy products from their diet. This is well worth your effort.

As well, I believe that Candida albicans yeast is rampant in children because of the over-use of antibiotics in our culture.

Children's symptoms and problems turn around miraculously when offending substances are removed from their diets and environment. It's a simple as that.

If you want "your child back," I urge you to focus on this area as quickly as possible.

You will have the best chance for dietary compliance when your children are little — before they are indoctrinated by television and the influences of other children.

Take sugar and dairy products out of the house — these are the biggest culprits.

Thankfully, grain allergies in children are much less prevalent unless they are obese. Then they are likely to be sensitive to wheat and flour-based products as well as corn.

Substitute honey, maple syrup and Stevia for sweeteners and use them very *sparingly*. These are sweets and they will have an effect on Candida overgrowth, but they will not have a significant effect on mood and behavior.

In place of dairy products, substitute soy milk (if tolerated), rice milk, almond milk or coconut milk. Some health food stores carry potato milk called vegimilk.

I recommend that these milks are used only for cereal (a healthy variety) or for making "smoothies." They are not necessary for drinking.

Because many alternative milks, contain sweeteners such as rice syrup and barley malt they should only be used in limited amounts. Some children thrive on goat's milk and goat's cheese.

The best drink, and one we need to teach children to get excited about, is WATER.

Place a large pitcher of water on the dinner table and make purified water accessible any time.

There are other sources of calcium besides milk: green leafy vegetables, nuts and whole grains. Calcium supplementation may be necessary.

SNACKS:

I suggest that you create a "snack cupboard" accessible to your child. Load up the cupboard with wholesome chips, healthy crackers, non-sugar fruit leather, pure juices or toasted nuts. Each child can pick 1 snack item at the appropriate time from this cupboard. Nut butters in place of peanut butter on whole grain crackers make a great snack. Soy cheese, cut up vegetables, chunks of protein and roasted nuts, set out on a tray make an appealing snack for the whole family. For picky eaters, a snack tray like this ensures your child is getting appropriate nutrition without the usual dinner time trials.

BREAKFAST:

Lets face it, most kids are addicted to cereal. Choose non-sugar cereals from the health food store, appropriate milks suggested above, a hand full of roasted nuts sprinkled on top with a few berries and a few tablespoons of coconut milk. Overweight children may respond more favorably to a protein based breakfast.

For sweetener, use powdered Stevia.

Eggs are a common allergen, especially for young children. Give your child adequate protein at breakfast: eggs (if not allergic), turkey sausage, turkey meatballs, turkey bacon, soy bacon etc. Toast or alternative bread — toasted.

LUNCH:

Hot lunches at school are a real problem. Macaroni and cheese (there's that dairy again) the "forced milk" program, gelatin, and all the rest of it. How are kids supposed to learn and behave on this junk?

With an overweight, highly allergic or behavior-problem child, carrying a sack lunch may be the only answer.

Sandwich with protein filling; almond butter and very light on *all-fruit* jelly; a small package of roasted/unsalted nuts; fruit for desert; bottled water* or pure juice to drink; cut up vegetables; cut up chunks of cold meat; soy cheese chunks; small bag of healthy chips.

DINNER:

Slow-cooker meals work well for busy families. Teach your child to help you in the kitchen. A six-year-old can make a salad and a much younger child can set the table.

Prepare a pot of steamed rice and a meal is created — with leftovers!

---

*Buy a non-leaching plastic bottle and re-use it. This will cut down on the mind-boggling amount of waste created by disposable plastic containers (even when recycled). Refill with purified water at home or at your local water store. No plastic bottle should be placed in direct sunlight.

DESSERTS:

No dessert is necessary after a hearty dinner. Save dessert for special occasions.

Fresh cut-up fruit or a fruit smoothie, are great choices.

SMOOTHIE:

1 cup fresh fruit

1 cup alternative milk or ½ cup water and ½ cup coconut milk

4 ice cubes

Blend at high speed for two minutes.

FROZEN BANANA:

When bananas are over-ripe, freeze them in a large ziplock bag. When needed, take one frozen banana, cut into chunks and blend at high speed. Sprinkle a little cinnamon or roasted carob on top and chopped toasted almonds. Remember one medium banana is approximately 25 grams of carbohydrate. If your child's weight reaches a plateau, watch carbohydrate grams.

PRETEND COOKIE:

1 rice cake or 2–4 rice crackers spread with nut butter and sprinkled with Stevia, roasted carob or cinnamon. 1 rice cake = 8–10 grams of carbohydrate. 1 rice

cracker = 2 grams of carbohydrate.

Spend time with your overweight child and exercise together. Buy a piece of gym equipment, post a training schedule and establish a "reward' incentive for daily exercise.

Chapter 18

Testing Yourself for Food Allergies

Pulse Testing

Wouldn't you like to know your own food allergies? There is simple method of testing the body for offending foods, beverages, and substances. It is called pulse testing. When I was first tested for all of my food allergies using P/N (provocation/neutralization testing), a process where allergens are injected under the skin, I was very aware of a raised pulse rate for certain substances. A raised pulse can indicate a potential "immune reaction" to a certain allergen thus contributing to unwanted symptoms.

We are going to use your pulse to test you for your own food allergies.

Begin by taking your *first two fingers* and placing them on the side of your neck so that you can feel the pulse in your carotid arteries. The carotid arteries are the main blood supply channels to your head. These pulse points on your neck should be easy to find and they will have a strong steady beat.

Get to know what a normal pulse in these areas feels like. You can also find a pulse in your temple point, at the right and about two inches above your eye. Try placing your fingers on the temple and feel the pulse of the blood flowing under the skin. Get to know what a normal pulse feels like in this area as well. You can also test your pulse in your wrist, although for some people, this may not be as easy to detect.

About twenty minutes after you have eaten or drunk anything, put your fingers on the pulse point that you are testing. If you have consumed something that is an allergy or sensitivity to the body, your pulse rate will increase, signifying that the body doesn't like what you have just consumed. This is called cardiac stimulation. The offending food has triggered an immune reaction and has signaled a message to the heart to increase the flow of blood through the arteries to dilute the toxins or poisons in the bloodstream.

At this point, noting your elevated pulse rate, just think and say to yourself, "What have I just eaten, drunk, or come in contact with that could be causing a reaction?" Now think back to what you had at your last meal and put your clues together. This helps to develop your own intuition about the foods that are right for your body. When you discover the offending substance, leave it out of your diet and *challenge* yourself (see below), again taking note of your increase in pulse rate. It usually takes between two to four hours, sometimes even longer, for the pulse rate to return to normal.

When people are aware of their food allergies, blood pressure can often return to normal levels.

Pulse testing is also useful to detect sensitivities to chemicals such as tobacco smoke, perfumes and cleaning compounds. If a person walks past you wearing perfume or you are pumping gas at a service station, and you are is sensitive to these items, an increased pulse rate can also be noted.

Challenge Testing

This is another type of testing which is easy, though somewhat time consuming. This is called a food *challenge*. Assuming that the most common allergies or sensitivities are caffeine, sugar, wheat, dairy (particularly milk) corn and soy, these are the main items you will want to focus on in your challenge. There are other common food sensitivities as well: eggs, tuna, citrus fruits and juices, certain fish, shellfish, nuts and spices. You may already be aware of sensitivities to these items.

Take all of these items out of your diet for 5–7 days to give the body a rest and to clear the system. Now, one item at a time, with a day of separation between each item, *challenge* yourself to the effects of each offending food. On an empty stomach, first thing in the morning, sit down to a very large portion of each food and nothing else. Half a cup of sugar on an empty stomach one morning, two cups of strong black coffee and nothing else the next morning, two pieces of whole wheat toast the next morning, two glasses of milk etc. Within 20 minutes of consuming your *challenge* food, if you are allergic or sensitive to it, there will be a reaction. You may notice that your heart pounds, your pulse may race, your stomach doubles up in knots, you have intestinal gas, you develop a headache etc. Note your reactions and take this item out of your diet. This is an offending food. Then carry on and eat the rest of your meals, which do not contain sensitive items. You have done your research. Your body knows, and it is showing you how to become more intuitive.

Your desire is to understand your body from an emotional and physical perspective. The body is not just a moving mass of flesh and bone. It is an elegant and complex set of systems, which, when given the right elements in the right combination, according to its directives, will function optimally for a lifetime.

Now let's focus on how you are going to eat on a daily basis. Rather than lay out elaborate meals, I prefer to give you guide lines for breakfast, lunch and dinner, snacks, traveling and eating out as well as entertaining. This I call "*The Body Knows Diet* Food Plan," which applies to people who want to lose weight as well as those who want to stop symptoms caused by immune system reactions.

Chapter 19

The Body Knows Diet
Food Plan

The following is a basic, easy-to-follow plan.

- Use whole, fresh, organic foods where possible.
- Read labels.
- Eat the foods that your body really wants. The idea with a plan such as this is to keep it simple. You don't have to take things down to the "last gnat's eyebrow," or the last degree, as far as foods are concerned. What you are trying to do is to avoid sugars, caffeine, and the common food allergens, give your digestive and immune system a rest, and feed yourself healthy, satisfying meals. Always drink six to eight glasses of purified or spring water per day.
- If you are trying to lose weight, reduce your carbohydrates.

- This plan is not designed for children.
- If you are pregnant or lactating, consult your doctor before starting any program.
- I like to keep my carbohydrates low. That way I have consistent energy and mental clarity. This is the way I eat.

Breakfast

- Eggs any style — often omelet-style with chopped, steamed vegetables such as cauliflower, broccoli, zucchini, ½ a carrot for color, green beans etc. Cook and drain the vegetables first before adding the beaten eggs. Add salt and pepper and spices or herbs as desired.
- Eggs can be an allergen for some people. This sensitivity can manifest as nausea, headaches, digestive problems, rashes, or mood changes. Because eggs are created through a hen's reproductive system, they are a hormone component. I have actually seen people break down and cry when they were injected with egg extract during allergy testing in a clinical setting. Most people are aware of their allergy to eggs.

Some breakfast alternatives

- Organic turkey sausages, chicken sausages or salmon, poultry, or meat from the previous night's dinner, with or without steamed vegetables. If you are not allergic to soy or beans, try a tofu and vegetable scramble.

- Breakfast on-the-run might be 2 Wasa (whole rye) crackers with almond butter.
- I do not eat fruit with my breakfast. I occasionally have fruit during the day or after dinner, several hours after a meal. I feel better, have more energy, mental clarity, stamina, and no food cravings if I stay away from carbohydrates at breakfast and lunch. On the weekends, if I am at home, I enjoy a slice of 100% rye toast with my breakfast. Because I have a wheat (flour) sensitivity, I stay away from it where possible. Wheat in any form makes me tired and frequent exposures to wheat make my joints stiff.

Drinks
- Herbal tea or coffee substitute with a drop of natural sugar substitute (stevia). No dairy products. Drink plenty of water.

Lunch
- A large salad composed of a variety of interesting lettuce plus chopped green vegetables of any sort. (Some people are sensitive to the cabbage or Mustard Food Family: broccoli, cauliflower,

cabbage, Brussels sprouts, kale etc. These vegetables can cause digestive problems such as discomfort, gas or burping. Check the *Food Family* list on p. 221 for alternatives.)

Next, add any of the following "goodies" into your salad, such as: red pepper (watch tomatoes — many people are sensitive to the acid in this fruit/vegetable), toasted sunflower seeds, chopped olives, avocado, marinated artichoke hearts, marinated cold vegetables from last night's dinner, cubed cold chicken or turkey, chunks of cold salmon, beef, lamb, or (if not allergic) beans (garbanzos are delicious), or tofu. On occasion I add canned salmon to the salad. Canned tuna can become an allergy because people consume it so frequently. Fresh tuna, which is rarely consumed, is usually non-allergic.

I like to sprinkle the top of my salad with goat feta cheese or sheep cheddar or sheep Romano cheese. Dairy products made from cow's milk cause me to experience fluid retention, puffy eyes, blocked eustachian tubes, post-nasal drip, and mild deafness in my left ear. Because sheep and goat products are a different food family and are not from a cow, they usually do not trigger histamine reactions in dairy sensitive people. Check to see if your nose runs or you retain fluid from sheep or goat milk products. Check the food family list on page 221. Butter is a dairy product. But because butter contains very *few* milk solids, which can trigger immune reactions, it is usually permissible.

Remember — eggs are not dairy products.

- Sometimes when I don't feel like chopping a bunch of vegetables, I make *roll ups* by placing my protein selection in a large lettuce leaf or cabbage leaf and rolling it up. Roll-ups can be made more exotic by adding any of the vegetables or ingredients from the list above. Thinly sliced ham or turkey slices can also be used as a basis for roll-ups.

Occasionally I enjoy two buttered Wasa (whole rye) crackers with my lunch. But I usually stay away from carbohydrates with this meal also. I find that I have better energy that way.

Dressings

- Use any oil and vinegar dressing. Even if you are eradicating Candida yeast and ferments should be avoided, vinegar in small amounts should be permissible. Sensitivity to ferments usually manifests in nasal congestion, a runny nose, post nasal drip, or headaches.
- People who are not sensitive to citrus fruits (lemon, orange, and grapefruit) may use lemon or lime juice in place of vinegar in salad dressings. Remember to stay away from

dressings containing sugar and dairy products. Ranch dressing contains cream, and Caesar salad dressing contains cream and cheese. Read labels. Add mayonnaise to your dressing to make it creamy. Mayonnaise is made from eggs and oil. It does not contain dairy products.

- When I am at home, I like to make my own dressing.

3 tbsp flax seed oil (high in essential fatty acids) or olive oil.
1 tsp vinegar — apple cider, balsamic, or rice wine variety.
1/2 tsp creamy Dijon mustard.
Pinch of coarse, Celtic sea salt.
Fresh ground pepper.

In place of Dijon mustard, I use fresh herbs such as chopped basil, dill, or parsley.

As an alternative flavor, I use sesame seeds, fresh ginger, and 1 tsp soy sauce or soy sauce alternative.

Shake well in a glass jar and serve over salad.

Mid-afternoon snack

- Enjoy a handful of roasted, unsalted nuts* with a cup of herbal tea.

  This protein snack boosts energy and sustains me until dinner. Be sure the nuts are roasted. I

---

* People with nut allergies are usually well aware of their sensitivities. Substitute other protein for a snack.

roast them myself. Place nuts on a cookie sheet in an oven preheated to 250° for approximately ½ hour or until golden brown. There is nothing more delicious than a pan of freshly roasted nuts. Raw nuts often contain mold, which can be a problem for people with mold allergies.

- Whole rye crackers, rice cakes, or rice crackers (found in the oriental section of most grocery stores) spread with almond, cashew, hazelnut or macadamia nut butter, and a cup of herbal tea sweetened with natural sweetener. Seed butters are also tasty. Remember that peanuts are a common allergy. Peanuts are legumes (beans).
- ½ apple thinly sliced and dipped in nut or seed butter.

  ½ apple contains 8 grams of carbohydrate. (Carbohydrate grams in fruit mount up quickly)

  ¼ cup almonds or cashews or 1 tbsp nut butter contain 8 grams of carbohydrate.
- 2 celery stalks filled with almond or cashew nut butter.
- 2 ham, beef or salami slices rolled around a chunk of cucumber or a chunk of *goat* feta cheese or sheep cheddar.
- 2 devilled eggs.

Dinner

- Eat any vegetable cooked or raw and any animal or vegetable protein source to which you are not allergic. Choose vegetable that are low in carbohydrate and eat plenty of them. See vegetable choices on page 122. I find that most people do better and feel more stable with animal protein. Try my delicious turkey meatball recipe on the next page.

  Along with your protein and vegetable choice, add any non-allergic carbohydrate. If you are trying to lose weight and watching carbohydrate grams, remember that 1 medium potato = 20 grams, ½ cup cooked rice = 20 grams, 1 ear of corn = 20 grams.

- Many people have poor absorption through the G.I. tract or stomach problems do not seem to tolerate grains well. As an alternative, to give the digestive system a rest, try using starchy vegetables such as squash, sweet potatoes or yams in place of grains for a few weeks. Instinctively, you will know whether grains or these starchy vegetables are easier for you to digest. I usually have a very small amount of squash (yellow winter, butternut, or Danish) with my dinner.

- You will find that taking digestive enzymes with each meal really helps your body to break down proteins, and aids in absorption and assimilation. Helps with gas and bloating, too! Digestive enzymes are available at the health-food store.

Turkey Meatballs

2 stalks celery — finely chopped
1 medium carrot — finely chopped
1 tsp "Spike" herbal seasoning mix (available at health food stores)
1 lb. ground turkey
1 tbsp Braggs Aminos, non-fermented soy sauce (health food store item), or soy sauce
Combine chopped celery, carrots and Spike.
Sauté until soft in 1 tbsp olive oil.
Mix Bragg's Aminos, and ground turkey
Add cooked celery and carrots
Form into balls.
Fry meatballs in olive oil until golden brown
Great for breakfast, any meal, and as a hot or cold snack
Travel well in an insulated bag. Freeze well too.
Kids love them!

- Eat slowly and enjoy your meal. Treat yourself to a beautiful table setting and pleasant surroundings while eating. Teach your children how to respect their bodies and eat in this way.

- Wait 20 minutes after your meal to allow the *good-feeling* brain chemical serotonin to be released. Most people do not feel hungry after such a meal. After 20 minutes, if you are still hungry, go back and have *more dinner*.

- After dinner, brew a cup of herbal tea, coffee substitute or decaffeinated coffee unless you are legume sensitive (coffee is a bean and a legume). Drink it unsweetened or if you need that sweet taste, add a drop of natural sweetener (Stevia), which is available at health food stores. Often just the very taste of a sweetener, even a natural sweetener, can evoke a need for *more* sweet!

- If you are disciplined (note the word *disciplined*), and a small amount of sweet won't derail your program, then try a piece (1-inch square) of *pecan coconut crunch* listed below, which may be useful as a dessert.

COCONUT PECAN CRUNCH
Makes about 2 dozen squares; approx. 8 grams
carbohydrate per square

1 cup butter
2 Tbsp honey or 1 tsp Stevia or to taste (natural herb sweetener)
1 tsp pure vanilla extract
3 tbsp powdered carob

½ to 1 cup toasted pecans, walnuts, or a mixture of favorite nuts.

¼ cup shredded unsweetened coconut (optional)

- Grease a 9" square baking pan or 9" pie plate. Line the bottom of the pan with roasted nuts and coconut.
- Melt butter over very low heat add honey, vanilla and carob. Pour this mixture over the nuts and coconut.
- Place directly in freezer. Stir several times while cooling to prevent butter from rising to the top. In approximately ½ hour when solid, cut and serve. (This treat needs to be stored frozen.) It is very rich. Enjoy one piece after dinner with a cup of herbal tea.
- This recipe is not suitable for people who have nut allergies or who are sensitive to some varieties of beans.

- Another choice for an after dinner treat could be one third of a high-protein, low- carbohydrate bar purchased from a health food store.
- Be careful, many of these bars contain ingredients to which you might be allergic, such as whey (found in dairy products) cocoa, soy beans or peanuts (beans/ legumes) as well as additives and chemicals.

- • For most people, a third of a bar should not trigger reactions but research this for yourself. I am not a big fan of these bars. I feel that for the most part, they are for emergency use only — when stuck in an airport or bivouacked at the side of a road, or on a long hike. But for many people the transition away from sweets is very difficult and some allowable sweet becomes an important lifeline. Fresh fruit can be a welcome after-dinner choice. Best: no dessert at all.

- • I reserve sweet desserts to the times when I am having dinner out with friends and something homemade or very special will tempt me. Usually after such an exposure I will feel "off," tired, or have that hung-over feeling the next day. When I am working or speaking it is not worth the price of having such a treat.

Options

This way of eating is always a pleasure. Think of eating like a prince or princess. Choose wholesome, even expensive ingredients. Actually your food bill will probably decline when you are not purchasing expensive packaged items. Use olive oil when sautéing vegetables or meats. Use cold marinated vegetables as a change from, or an addition to, salads. Save leftover vegetables to add them to a morning omelet. Experiment with fresh ginger, fresh herbs, and spices. Treat yourself well. *Cook!* Some people actually find they are cooking for the first time — and really enjoying it.

Treat yourself well. **Cook!**

I remember a consultation with a woman who lived in a large American city, famous for its glitz, glamour, and fancy restaurants. When I broached the subject of cooking to her, she was horrified, exclaiming that she never cooked, but purchased all her meals and beverages in restaurants. When I asked her if she had a stove, she paused for a moment and admitted that although she had lived in her current residence for five years, she had never used the stove!

For people like these, I recommend the use of a **slow cooker** or a **table-top-grill**. A slow-cooker works very well and is a lazy way to prepare an evening meal — eight hours ahead — in the morning.

- Take any sort of meat you wish to cook. Chicken, turkey or beef works well. Lamb shanks are wonderfully tasty cooked in a crock-pot. Place the meat in the crock-pot and add approximately two cups of water, stock, chicken or beef broth. Season to taste with salt, pepper, fresh herbs, or non-fermented soy sauce. Add a chopped onion, two chopped celery stalks, and a chopped carrot. Add ½ cup red wine. The alcohol evaporates in cooking, and the rich flavor is delicious.

- Turn on the slow cooker and leave to simmer for the day. Eight hours later you will return to delicious smells and an inviting meal. Cook a pot of rice or a baked potato and fix a quick salad and voilà! The evening meal is prepared and there are plenty of leftovers.

- Another convenient way to cook is with a **table-top-grill**. The grill is about the size of a tennis racquet and sits at an angle on the kitchen counter so that the fat from the meat drips down into a container below the grill. Place any meat you wish to cook on the surface of the hot grill — chicken breasts, turkey sausages, steak or lamb chops work well. Brush the surface of the meat with non-fermented soy sauce and sprinkle with herbs or spices. Then arrange cut-up vegetables next to the meat — eggplant slices, zucchini strips, or peppers etc. After 10–15 minutes, turn the meat over and grill the other side. Remove the vegetables. Serve this meal with any appropriate starch or carbohydrate of your choice.

The body knows that it is loved. As you prepare your foods with love and care, this energy is positively transmitted to body parts and processes.

The body knows that it is loved. As you prepare your foods with love and care, this energy is positively transmitted to body parts and processes.

Eating out

- Eating in restaurants doesn't need to be difficult. Your best choices are steak or seafood restaurants, Chinese, Thai or Indian restaurants offer interesting flavors and minimal exposures to wheat and dairy products. Italian restaurants are usually off limits unless you can pick your way through the bread, pasta and cheese. Recently on a trip to Tuscany, I was able to completely avoid wheat and dairy products by choosing the protein and vegetable choices at meals as well as marvelous salads made from fresh garden greens, steamed fennel laced with olive oil, fresh basil and balsamic vinegar.

- In restaurants, you can always order rice or a baked potato with dinner if you are sensitive to wheat. Remember to count carbohydrate grams. Most baked potatoes are large enough for 2 people. Potatoes convert from starch to sugar very easily. So order just a very few home fries or hash browns in place of toast at breakfast.

- Salads and steamed vegetables are always available. Salad bars offer you control over portions and choices. Order vegetables without cheese or sauce, which often contains dairy products. Order oil and vinegar or a vinaigrette dressing with salads, thus avoiding dressings, like ranch or blue cheese dressing that contain dairy products.

- Eggs, chicken, turkey, fish, shellfish, lamb, beef, pork, beans, and legumes are all good protein choices. A favorite of mine is my protein of choice — a steak, lamb, fish or seafood, and double vegetables — keep the carbs low and skip the rice or potato.

- Ask about the ingredients of sauces and dressings. If in doubt order it on the side and trust your instincts regarding amounts to take. Tofu, unless you are in a vegetarian or Asian restaurant, is rarely on the menu.

- I rarely eat beans, which, though high in protein and well tolerated by many people, are also high in carbohydrate. Beans upset my digestive system and give me gas — not great when working with the public. Tofu is made from soybeans. Soy is a common allergen, has an estrogenic effect and may increase estrogen levels. High estrogen levels have been linked to breast cancer and other estrogen-related cancers.

- Some forms of animal protein are more digestible than others — fish or lamb are usually tolerated.
- Carry a bag of herbal tea with you. Most restaurants carry a selection of herbal teas or will bring you a mug of hot water and lemon.

Traveling

- I always carry nuts (usually roasted almonds) with me when I travel. I also carry a selection of protein bars. These can be a lifesaver if I am starving and a flight is delayed or if I arrive at a hotel late at night. Other than emergency situations, I am not in favor of protein bars because they usually contain additives or offending foods. There is rarely food that I can eat on an airplane. I will pick away at what is offered and fill in with nuts. Often I will carry cold meat slices, turkey meat balls and chunks of celery or cucumber in a small, insulated bag. These need to be consumed within several hours of leaving home.
- I always carry a package of Ry Krisp or Wasa (100% rye) crackers with me. Having these on hand helps me to avoid wheat and its subsequent ill effects. I also carry a small, plastic, screw-top container of cashew nut or almond butter, sealed in a plastic bag. This I liberally coat on the Wasa crackers for a fast breakfast or late night snack.

- I like to choose hotels with a refrigerator in my room. I ask a friend in the city I am visiting to stock the refrigerator with a selection of vegetables, hardboiled eggs, and cold meats and poultry. I draw from this supply while I am working during the day. I usually enjoy a meal with friends or a restaurant dinner at night.

- When I am exposed to sweet desserts or a glass of wine, I use my intuition and I ask how many bites of a sweet dessert I should take before my body will react to fluctuating blood sugar levels. The answer might be two bites or six bites, depending on the item. After the intuited number-of-bites are consumed, I put down my fork. If I exceed my intuited limit, I will invariably feel "off" the next day.

- When it comes to wine, I am acutely aware of my limits and therefore drink wine very occasionally, probably once or twice a month on average. I approach the glass of wine in the same way, tuning into the beverage and sensing the amount that would be "enough." I find that about six sips is my limit. Wine is a powerful stimulant; a small amount will change my body chemistry and alter my personality. But on occasion, I like the buzz that wine gives me as well as its relaxing effects. I also find that I get less dehydrated if I take one sip of wine and four sips of water in between, alternating in this manner until my designated number of sips is finished. Then I look at the glass of wine and know that it is time to switch to sparkling water with a slice of lemon or lime. With this approach I tolerate these items in small amounts.

- Discipline in food consumption is an important level of personal mastery. Foods are chemicals and medicines. When we feel good physically there are benefits which are felt on the emotional and spiritual levels as well.

> *Discipline in food consumption is an important level of personal mastery.*

- When you are starting a food program, keep everything as simple as possible. Don't try and get fancy or complicated, like trying to make fancy sauces out of alternative and exotic types of flour. Avoid the sauces and the strain on yourself and within 30 days enjoy the occasional sauce in a restaurant or at a friend's home. This is not the time to be making angel food cakes out of mung bean flour. You will be back to eating *real* angel food cake again on a very occasional basis after you have spent a few weeks clearing your body of toxins and histamine reactions. If you are cooking for a family, cook normally for them, and stick to your program. Enjoy: this is a life- and health-changing experience.

Daily Food Diary

The following are food diary sheets that you can fill in every day. Try and make your notations after each meal so that you are aware of what you are eating, how well you are doing as you avoid offending foods.

Be sure to complete the section on the right hand side of the sheet noting down reactions to any foods and also the benefits of your new program such as: less bloating, rings seem looser, stomach feels calmer, less headaches etc.

Make additional copies of the diary and fill them out faithfully each day until your routine is well-established — usually in 30 days. For menu ideas, refer to "*The Body Knows Diet* Food Plan" on page 191, and the recipes contained in "*The Body Knows*" *Cookbook*.

Find a "buddy" or friend to check in with on a daily basis. You can motivate each other, swap recipes and share in the excitement of following *The Body Knows Diet*.

My Food & Progress Log

Day/Date _____

Meal	# Carb. Grams	Offending Foods Consumed Y/N	Allergic Reaction Y/N	Exercise Y/N	Weight Gained/ Fluid Retained Y/N	Energy/Well-Being Observations
Breakfast						
Snack						
Lunch						
Snack						
Dinner						
Snack						

Supplementation

Along with your food program, I recommend that you also take supplements. I prefer whole food supplements rather than synthesized or laboratory produced supplements. The body takes its nutrition from food, not from man-made supplements. I think that people are taking far too many supplements. They are trying to boost their energy and reduce their symptoms by taking copious amounts of vitamins when they can gain more energy and nutrition from eating the right foods.

I take:

Digestive enzymes — this helps the stomach to break down proteins and digest and absorb nutrients from your food.

Multiple Vitamin/Mineral Combination — a plant-based multiple vitamin that contains all the nutrients derived from whole food sources.

Calcium — calcium derived from plants may be more easily assimilated than synthesized calcium.

Vitamin C — 500 mg daily — also derived from whole foods.

Cod Liver Oil — 1 tablespoon per day

As well as the regimen above, I take an anti-Candida supplement on a regular basis and I work closely with my endocrinologist on hormone balance. I drink eight glasses of filtered water, get eight hours of sleep each night and exercise moderately every day. I am energetic and I feel and look much younger than my 60 years.

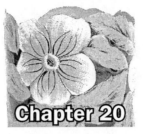

Chapter 20

Personal Motivation

The time has come to turn the helm over to you. I have given you the tools now it's up to you to use them. You have a rich, rewarding life ahead of you. Your family, your friends and loved ones are all counting on you to be here healthy and strong to fulfill your destiny and live the life you have dreamed of having. Happiness, optimism and well being are dependent on a healthy body functioning at its ideal weight. Why wait — there is nothing to lose but those unwanted pounds. The body "knows," and it will support you and reflect back to you all the positive steps you are taking. You have my every blessing and good wish for continued success toward your goal.

CARBOHYDRATE GRAM COUNTER

Food	Amount	Carbo. Grams
ANIMAL PROTEIN		
Chicken, Beef, Fish,		0
Lamb, Turkey, Veal, Pork,		
(Ham, Bacon)		0
Shellfish, Wild Meats, Eggs		0
DAIRY PRODUCTS		
Whole milk	1 cup	12
Ice cream	½ cup	15
Cheese	1 oz hard	1
Cottage cheese	½ cup	4
Sour cream	1 tbsp	1
Yogurt	½ cup	8
FATS		
Butter	1 tbsp.	0
French dressing	1 tbsp.	2
Vegetable oil	unlimited	0
Olive oil	unlimited	0
Mayonnaise	1 tbsp.	0

(continued)

Food	Amount	Carbo. Grams
NUTS		
Mixed	¼ cup	5
Almonds	¼ cup	5
Peanut butter	2 tbsp	5
Cashew nut butter	2 tbsp	11
VEGETABLES		
Alfalfa sprouts (raw)	½ cup	
Arugula	unlimited	0
Artichoke	1 medium	14
Asparagus	10 spears	4
Beans, green.	1 cup cooked	8
Beets	1 cup cooked	6
Broccoli	1 cup cooked	5
Brussels sprouts	6	5
Cabbage	1 cup shredded, raw	3
Cabbage	1 cup cooked	5
Carrots	1 medium, raw	5
Carrots	1 cup cooked	12
Cauliflower	1 cup	4
Celery	2 stalks	2
Corn	1 ear	20
Cucumber	1 medium	6
Eggplant	1 cup cooked	6
Kale	1 cup cooked	3
Lettuce	unlimited	0
Okra	1 cup	11
Onions	½ cup, raw	5
Onions	½ cup cooked	10
Green peas	1 cup	20
Green pepper	1 large	5
Potatoes	1 small	20
Spinach	1 cup cooked	4
Squash	1 cup cooked	10

Food	Amount	Carbo. Grams
Tomatoes	1 medium	4
Turnip	½ cup	8
Ketchup	1 tbsp.	5
Tomato juice	1 cup	5

BEANS (LEGUMES)

Food	Amount	Carbo. Grams
Tofu	½ cup	20
Lima beans	½ cup	25
Kidney beans	½ cup	13
White beans	½ cup	22
Fava beans	½ cup	16
Soy flour	½ cup	12

FRUIT

Food	Amount	Carbo. Grams
Apples	1 large	20
Apricots	4	14
Avocado	½	5
Banana	1 medium	25
Strawberries	1 cup	7
Raspberries	1 cup	8
Blackberries	1 cup	10
Blueberries	1 cup	17
Cantaloupe	1 cup	12
Grapefruit	½ small	8
Grapes	½ cup	8
Lemons	1 medium	8
Lime	1 medium	8
Orange	1 small	11
Orange juice	1 cup	22
Peach	1 medium	8
Pear	1 medium	20
Pineapple	1 cup	17
Pineapple	½ cup, canned	18

Food	Amount	Carbo. Grams
Plum	1 large	18
Watermelon	1 cup	11

BREADS & CEREALS

Food	Amount	Carbo. Grams
Bagel	1	27
Bread	1 slice	20
Hamburger bun	1	23
English muffin	1	25
Pita round	1	20
Rice cake	1	8
Rice crackers	2	4
Saltine cracker	1	2
Wasa (rye) cracker	1	7
Cornflakes	1 cup	17
Oatmeal	1 cup cooked	20
Shredded wheat	1 large	23
Spaghetti, macaroni, pasta	1 cup	25–30
Noodles (egg)	1 cup	26
Rice	1 cup cooked	20

SWEETENERS

Food	Amount	Carbo. Grams
Honey	1 tbsp	15
White sugar	1 tsp	4
Brown sugar	1 tbsp.	10
Stevia (herb sweetener)	1 tsp	1
Syrup	1 tbsp.	15

SPIRITS

Food	Amount	Carbo. Grams
Wine (red or white)	1 glass	3
Light Beer	8 oz	4

For a complete list of carbohydrate grams, refer to *Protein Power*, Eades (Bantam).

FOOD FAMILIES

The following is a list of common food families. When avoiding *offending* foods, it can be helpful to check the food family list and avoid foods that are in the same family.

* = Single food families.

PLANTS

APPLE
Apple
Apple Cider
Pear
Pectin
Quince & Seed
Vinegar

BAMBOO*
Shoots

BANANA
Arrowroot
Banana
Plantain

BARLEY
Malt

BEET
Beet
Beet Sugar
Chard
Lamb Quarters
Spinach
Thistle

BIRCH
Filbert
Hazelnut
Wintergreen

BRAZIL NUT*
Brazil Nut

BUCKWHEAT
Buckwheat
Garden sorrel
Rhubarb

CACTUS
Cactus
Prickly Pear
Tequila

CANE
Sugar
Molasses

CAPER*
Capers

CARROT
Carrots
Celeriac
Celery

Coriander
Cumin
Dill
Fennel
Parsley
Parsnip

CASHEW
Cashew
Mango
Pistachio

CHICORY*

CITRUS
Angostura
Citron
Grapefruit
Kumquat
Lemon
Lime
Orange
Tangerine

COCOA BEAN
Cocoa
Cocoa chocolate
Cola bean

COMPOSITE
Artichoke
Dandelion
Endive
Escarole
Jerusalem
   artichoke
Lettuce
Sesame oil
Sesame seed
Sunflower oil
Sunflower seed

CORN
Dextros
   (Glucose)
Meal
Oil
Starch
Sugar
Syrup

EBONY
Persimmon

FUNGI
Baker's yeast
Brewer's yeast
Mold
Mushroom

GINGER
Cardamom
Ginger
Turmeric

GOOSEBERRY
Currant
Gooseberry

GOURD
Casaba
Cantaloupe
Cucumber
Gherkin
Honeydew
Muskmelon
Persian melon
Pumpkin
Squash
Watermelon

GRAPE
Brandy
Champagne
Cream of tartar
Grapes
Raisin
Wine
Wine vinegar

HEATH
Blueberry
Cranberry
Huckleberry

IRIS
Saffron

LAUREL
Avocado
Bay leaves
Cinnamon
Sassafras

LILY
Aloes
Asparagus
Chives
Garlic
Leek
Onion
Sarsaparilla

LEGUMES
Black-eyed pea
Carob
Green pea
Jack bean
Kidney bean
Lecithin
Lentil
Licorice
Lima bean
Navy bean
Peanut and oil
Pinto
Senna
Soybean
Soy oil
Soy flour
String bean
Tonka bean

MADDER*
Coffee

MALLOW
Cottonseed meal
Cottonseed oil
Okra (Gumbo)

MAPLE
Maple sugar
Maple syrup

MILLET*

MINT
Basil
Horehound
Marjoram
Mint
Oregano
Peppermint
Sage
Spearmint
Thyme

MORNING GLORY
Sweet potato
Yam

MULBERRY
Breadfruit
Fig
Hop
Mulberry

MUSTARD
Broccoli
Cabbage
Cauliflower
Chinese cabbage
Collard
Horseradish
Kale
Kohlrabi

Kraut
Mustard
Mustard greens
Mustard seeds
Radish
Rape (canola)
Rutabaga
Sprouts
Swedes
Turnips
Watercress

MYRTLE
Allspice
Cloves
Guava
Paprika
Pimento

NIGHTSHADE
Belladonna
Black pepper
Chili pepper
Green pepper
Eggplant
Potato
Red cayenne
Red capsicum
Red pepper
Tobacco
Tomato
White pepper

NUTMEG
Mace
Nutmeg

OAK
Chestnut

OATS*

OLIVE
Black olives
Green olives
Olive oil

ORCHID*
Vanilla

PALM
Coconut
Date
Palm cabbage
Sago

PARSLEY
Anise
Angelica
Caraway
Celery
Celery seed
Carrots
Celeriac
Coriander
Cumin
Dill
Fennel
Parsley
Parsnips

PAWPAW
Pawpaw
Papain
Papaya

PINE
Juniper
Pinion Nut

PINEAPPLE*

POMEGRANATE*

POPPY*
Poppy seeds

PLUM
Almond
Apricot
Cherry
Nectarine
Peach
Plum
Prune
Wild cherry

RICE*

RYE*

ROSE
Blackberry
Boysenberry
Dewberry
Loganberry
Raspberry
Strawberry
Youngberry

SOAPBERRY
Lichi Nut

TAPIOCA*

TEA*

WALNUT
Black walnut
English walnut
Hickory nut
Pecan

WHEAT
Bran
Farina
Flour
Gluten Flour
Wheat germ
Whole wheat

WILD RICE*

MEAT
-Butter
-Cheese
-Gelatin

BIRDS
Chicken
Chicken eggs
Duck
Duck eggs
Goose
Goose eggs
Guinea hen
Grouse
Partridge
Pheasant
Squab

Turkey
Turkey eggs

FISH*

CRUSTACEANS
Crab
Crayfish
Lobster
Shrimp

MAMMALS
Beef
-butter
-cheese
-gelatin
-milk
-veal
Buffalo
Goat
-milk
-cheese
-mutton
Lamb
Pork
-bacon
-ham
Rabbit
Venison

MOLLUSKS
Abalone
Clam
Mussel
Oyster
Scallop
Snail
Squid

HIDDEN FOOD SOURCES

You may be surprised to find that your favorite foods are hiding out in the most unlikely places. This list can help you to identify *offending* foods, which could be hidden in other products. Read labels and get to know the ingredients of common, combination foods.

EGG
Baking powders
Bavarian cream
Breaded foods
Breads
Cake flours
Cakes
Custards
Eggs
French toast
Fritters
Frostings
Frying batters
Griddle cakes
Hamburger
  patties
Hollandaise
  sauce
Ice cream
Icings
Macaroni
Macaroons
Marshmallows
Mayonnaise
Meat loaf
Meringues
Noodles
Pancakes
Puddings
Rolls
Salad dressings
Sauces
Sausages
Soufflés
Waffles

YEAST
Beer
Bovril
Brandy
Breads
Buns
Cakes
Cereals
Cheeses
Chocolate
Condiments
Cookies
Crackers
French dressing
Fruit juices
Gin
Horseradish
Malted milk
Mayonnaise
Olives
Pastries
Pickles
Pretzels
Rolls
Rum
Sauerkraut
Soy sauce
Tomato sauce
Truffles
Vinegar
Vitamins
Vodka
Whiskey
Wine

WHEAT
Bagels
Biscuits
Bologna
Bread
Breaded
  meats/fish

Cakes
Cereals
Cookies
Corn bread
Crackers
Doughnuts
Dumplings
Flour
Gravies
Hot cakes
Liverwurst
Lunch meats
Macaroni
Pasta
Pie crust

SOYBEANS
Baby foods
Biscuits
Breads
Butter substitute
Cakes
Cereals
Cooking spray
Crackers
Hard candies
Ice cream
Lecithin
Lunch meats
Margarine
Mayonnaise
Milk substitute
Oils
Oriental sauces
Pastries
Salad dressings
Soups

Soy flour
Soy noodles
Tempura
Textured
  vegetable
  protein
Tofu

MILK
Biscuits
Breads
Buttermilk
Cakes
Cheese
Cheese dishes
Chocolate milk
Chowders
Cookies
Creamed foods
Custards
Fritters
Gravies
Ice cream
Malted cocoa
Mashed potatoes
Omelets
Ovaltine
Pancakes
Pancake mix
Potatoes,
  scalloped
Powdered milk
Salad dressing,
  creamy
Sherbets
Soda crackers
Soufflés

Soups, creamed
Sour cream
Waffles
Whey
Yogurt

CORN
All baked goods
Aspirin
Baking powder
Beer, ales
Biscuits
Breads, pastries
Butter substitute
Cakes, cookies
Candies
Carbonated
  beverages
Catsup
Chewing gum
Cornmeal
Corn oil
Cough syrups
Cream pies
Cured hams
Custard
Doughnuts
Graham
  crackers
Gravies
Grits
Gummed papers
Instant teas
Margarine
Non-dairy
  creamers
Pancake mix

Pie Crusts
Popcorn
Puddings,
 instant
Salad dressing

Sandwich
 spreads
Sausages
Soups, creamed
Stamp glue

Starch
Toothpaste
Tortillas
Whiskey

Weight-Loss Products

In order for your program to be successful, I have chosen specific products that are designed to enhance your body's ability to lose weight and your mind's ability to get behind your weight loss program.

1. *"The Body Knows" Diet —*
   Cracking the Weight-Loss Code $16.95
   (Including "Why Wait to Lose Weight" CD)

2. *"The Body Knows" Cookbook* $12.95

3. "Why Wait to Lose Weight" CD $14.95

4. "The Body Knows" DVD or VHS $19.95

5. Apa-Trol — Appetite Suppressant Drops
   (two-month supply) $22.00

6. Candida Yeast Eradication Supplement
   (120 capsules) $24.00

These items are available individually or as a package for $89.95 plus shipping and handling. Please order by fax to 360-527-3322.

Be sure to include your name, address, telephone number, Visa or MC number and expiration date plus a listing of the products you require.

These products are also available online when you sign up for the online weight loss program available through my Web site: www.thebodyknowsdiet.com

Online Weight-Loss Program

I'm excited to announce that "The Body Knows Diet" program is available online. Now you can participate in the program with me as I explain the five components of weight loss. You will feel part of a live audience, hear success stories and feel personally motivated not only to try "The Body Knows Diet" program, but to stick with it and experience success just as thousands of my clients have — without dieting, calorie counting, measuring or starving!

To view the online weight-loss program by video stream, visit my Web site at www.thebodyknowsdiet. com and click on "weight loss."

Suggested Reading

The Body "Knows" — *how to tune in to your body and improve your health,* by Caroline Sutherland

"The Body Knows" Cookbook, By Caroline Sutherland

The Yeast Connection Handbook, by William Crook, M.D.

Is This Your Child? Discovering and Treating Unrecognized Allergies in Adults and Children — Doris Rapp, M.D.

Protein Power, by Michael and Mary Dan Eades, M.D.

Your Hidden Food Allergies are Making You Fat: the ALCAT Food Sensitivities Weight Loss Breakthrough — Rudy Rivera M.D., and Roger D. Deutsch

Natural Hormone Balance — Uzzi Reiss, M.D.

What Your Doctor May Not Tell You About Menopause- John Lee, M.D.

The Schwarzbein Principle — Diana Schwarzbein M.D.

Sugar Busters — *Cut Sugar to Trim Fat* — Stewart, Andrews, Bethea, Balart

The No Grain Diet — Joseph Mercola M.D. www.mercola.com

Molecules of Emotion — Candace Pert, Ph.D.

You Can Heal Your Life — Louise L. Hay

Useful Reference:
Overeaters Anonymous
National Office
P.O. Box 00420
Rio Rancho, New Mexico
87174-4020
505-891-2664

Notes

Notes